Juju Sundin's

Birth*Skills*

with Sarah Murdoch

Proven pain-management techniques for your labour and birth

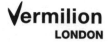

Vermilion
LONDON

7 9 10 8 6

Published in 2008 by Vermilion, an imprint of Ebury Publishing.
First published in Australia by Allen & Unwin Book Publishers in 2007.

Ebury Publishing is a Random House Group company.

The Random House Group Limited Reg. No. 954009

Addresses for companies within the Random House Group
can be found at www.randomhouse.co.uk

A CIP catalogue record for this book is available from the British Library

The Random House Group Limited supports The Forest Stewardship Council (FSC®), the
leading international forest certification organisation. Our books carrying the FSC label are
printed on FSC® certified paper. FSC is the only forest certification scheme endorsed by
the leading environmental organisations, including Greenpeace. Our paper procurement
policy can be found at www.randomhouse.co.uk/environment

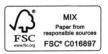

MIX
Paper from
responsible sources
FSC® C016897

Printed in the UK by CPI Group (UK) Ltd, Croydon, CR0 4YY

ISBN 9780091922146

Copies are available at special rates for bulk orders.
Contact the sales development team on 020 7840 8487 for more information.

To buy books by your favourite authors and register for offers, visit www.randomhouse.co.uk

The information in this book has been compiled by way of general guidance in
relation to the specific subjects addressed, but is not a substitute and not to be relied
on for medical, healthcare, pharmaceutical or other professional advice on specific
circumstances and in specific locations. Please consult your GP before changing,
stopping or starting any medical treatment. So far as the authors are aware the information
given is correct and up to date as at November 2007. Practice, laws and regulations all
change, and the reader should obtain up to date professional advice on any such issues.
The authors and publishers disclaim, as far as the law allows, any liability arising directly

Juju Sundin is a physiotherapist and has her own private obstetric

practi   with

pregn   and

motiv   style

has a   ome,

hospit   eeing

it as p   ls as

well a

J   s and

ignite   birth

skills   ng it

contr   and

Austr   tools

and te   used

by eve

H   d by

Sarah   rts of

how s

J

Sar   nally

as a n   ed to

philar   t not-

for-pr   table

assoc   ation,

the A   and a

direct

S   e is a

signif   preg-

nant with her first son she attempted to find a source that could educate
her about the physiology of labour and birth. Not finding anything satis-
factory in a book she attended Juju Sundin's birth skills classes. Sarah
credits her incredible birth experiences to Juju's skills and feels that
this knowledge should be passed on to all women.

Sarah lives in Sydney, Australia, with her husband Lachlan and her
two sons, Kalan and Aidan.

As always, this book is dedicated to my
two beautiful children Marina and Heidi.

Juju

To my two miracles, Kalan and Aidan,
and to my husband, Lachlan. I am truly blessed.

Sarah

CONTENTS

Foreword by Dr Keith Hartman   vii

Introduction Birth skills for life   ix
Birth skills   Your education starts now   1

Skills for the first stage of labour
Skill # 1   Movement   17
Skill # 2   Breathing and vocalising   51
Skill # 3   Visualisation   87
Skill # 4   Stress balls   113
Skill # 5   Keywords   139

Skills for the second stage of labour
Skill # 6   Pushing   169
Skill # 7   Crowning   189

Practice and preparation
Practice   Make sure you know your skills   209
Preparation   Posterior backache labour   223
Preparation   Medical help if you need it   239
Preparation   Motivation and birth skills   265

And finally ... The bigger picture   275

Acknowledgements   283
Index   285
Pregnancy and birth resources by Juju Sundin   290

Art completes what nature cannot seem to finish.

Aristotle

The art of childbirth completes what nature started and creates new meanings over time.

Juju Sundin

Foreword
Dr Keith Hartman

Over the past 30 years it has been my privilege and pleasure to be involved with the births of about 7,000 babies. It has been a great joy to share the excitement of those women's pregnancies and the exhilaration of their experience of birth. It has, however, been very obvious over that time that most women are really frightened of the prospect of labour.

Over the same period of time thousands of women have benefited from Juju Sundin's antenatal classes. Juju is an extraordinary person who is passionate about her subject and gifted in her ability to educate and inspire confidence. My patients have frequently told me of feeling empowered by her classes.

Juju is probably our most experienced and respected obstetric physiotherapist. Her unique strategies for understanding, embracing and dealing with the pain of labour are scientifically based and continually being refined. These strategies certainly work extremely well for many women. However, Juju's classes also educate women about all available options (including medical methods of pain relief) so that her clients do not feel locked into one approach to labour. She stresses that every person deals with pain differently and that no two labours are the same. Her classes include information about all the interventions that might prove necessary for the safety of the mother and her baby.

I find it interesting to reflect that when I was an obstetric registrar 30 years ago we had a few patients of various cultural backgrounds who were active and very noisy in labour. Their births were usually fast and straightforward and accompanied by tremendous emotional release. On the other hand most of our patients were expected to be much more passive. They were told to lie on the bed, not make a noise and to suffer the pain in silence, perhaps using some rehearsed breathing patterns for distraction from the pain. How pleasing it is that women are now being actively encouraged to express their feelings and reactions to labour in their own individual way. Mobility in labour certainly assists in the efficiency of uterine contractions. Vocalisation, visualisation, various distraction techniques and partner involvement all add to the positive experience of the process of childbirth.

Sarah Murdoch came to me as a patient and also attended Juju's classes. Her beautifully written pieces for this book will prove not only very interesting but also extremely valuable to the reader. Sarah has very honestly expressed her own initial fear of labour and the knowledge and self-confidence she obtained from Juju's tuition. I know she used the birth skills to great effect during her labour.

This excellent book will allow a much greater number of women to benefit from Juju Sundin's experience and expertise. Even her infectious enthusiasm is evident from the practical and easily understood way it is written.

Juju and Sarah's book should be read by anyone who believes that labour and childbirth are totally normal processes, which with education and support can be approached confidently and without fear. I congratulate them both on making such a valuable contribution to the preparation of women for birth – the most sublime and wondrous human experience.

Keith Hartman FRCOG, FRANZCOG
Visiting Specialist Obstetrician and Gynaecologist
  Royal North Shore Hospital, Sydney
  The Mater Hospital, North Sydney
  North Shore Private Hospital, St Leonards

INTRODUCTION

Birth skills for life

Sarah and I would like to welcome you to our book, which is designed to help you to prepare for the one thing all women worry about when having a baby: the pain of childbirth. We are going to help you to learn how to minimise the pain and, in doing so, we will educate you and empower you, so you can help yourself get through it.

Whether you are expecting a short labour, a long labour, a pain-free labour, a natural labour, an epidural-assisted labour, a water birth or even a labour similar to your mother's or sister's, the skills in this book will help you. Whether you are looking forward to labour, are ambivalent about it or are dreading it, these skills will help you. Even if you have an unexpected caesarean on the day, the information within these covers will still help you. In fact, even if you don't use our ideas for your child-birth, these techniques can be used as life skills. A number of my class participants have reported back to me about how they use the skills in other situations. One of my students told me she gives her 10-year-old daughter a stress ball to squeeze every time, say, a splinter needs to be taken out of her little foot! The technique works brilliantly, the mother said, and she learnt this skill in my classes over a decade ago.

Both Sarah and I have been through childbirth twice, but Sarah's first child and my last child are 25 years apart! Our joint contributions bring to you both a theoretical and an experiential perspective. We have written this book to make a difference and we hope, with both our hearts, that it does make a difference for you.

An evolving practice

I conducted my first antenatal class at the Royal Hospital for Women in Sydney on the day man landed on the moon, Monday 21 July 1969. Since then, the design of my classes has evolved and adapted to the changing needs of the women who attend them. I have seen all the antenatal trends come and go and, while respecting them all, I have fine-tuned my physio-therapy practice to concentrate on one thing and one thing only: mastering the pain of labour. My classes are not based on trends, but on basic factual anatomy, physiology, neurophysiology and human behav-iour. The evolution of my classes came about from years of me watching and learning and listening, of taking notice when someone told me some-thing mundane or something out of the ordinary about childbirth, of being awed by women's resilience during labour and never ridiculing any couple's way of coping, but rather being inspired by them. All of them.

I remember teaching the class on that momentous day back in 1969 and asking the women (partners did not attend then) how they felt about labour pain. They all looked at each other, shrugged their shoulders and laughed. They were simply resigned to the belief that it was 'just their lot to have to suffer the pain', there was nothing they could do about it. But if I arrived at my birth skill class tonight and posed exactly the same question to the group, not one would shrug their shoulders and laugh. Not one! That is not to say that the women today, nearly 40 years later, don't have a fear of the pain, but they are not prepared to be resigned to helplessness.

We now desire control over our experiences, much more so than our mothers and grandmothers did, and this is what drives most women to attend my classes. They want to know exactly what they can do during labour to handle the pain. They are seeking tools that will not go out the window on the day. Even though birth is not easy, mastering the pain is something that women can do with the skills in this book.

Choices in childbirth

I have a policy of supporting all methods of birth. I support all the women who pass through my practice no matter what sort of birth they have. I encourage them to make their own choices with their birth team, and that includes having the courage to choose an epidural if they need it, without feeling any sense of guilt. I think it's great that drugs and the medical team are there if you need them – I needed them myself, as did Sarah, as have some of the other women who attended my classes – but I also think there is something to be gained from equipping yourselves (and I mean the woman *and* her partner here) with knowledge and skills to take on some or all of the adventure of childbirth.

Many of you will already be excited about working through childbirth. Your decision about the birth may have already been made. May I suggest you be open to the medical system if you need it; there is much that you can control on the day, but there are also things that you can't. A healthy mother and baby is what childbirth is all about.

Having said that, I am asked over and over again why the rate of medication – from simple pain killers to epidurals and caesareans – during childbirth has gone through the roof. It has never been my style to critique doctors, hospitals or medical trends. I prefer to put passion and energy into trying to make a difference for women through my classes. I'm afraid, like it or not, it is we, the women, who are the ones asking for the drugs. It is as if we are so afraid of experiencing pain, we only feel calm and reassured when we know we can have it medically blocked out. We are so accomplished in our homes, hobbies, sports, relationships and careers, yet we are terrified of losing that same command in labour. So we, the women, are choosing drugs as a quick-fix, take-the-pain-away means of control.

Then again, many of our partners are also saying, 'Look, why don't you just have the drugs? It's crazy to feel pain when you don't have to!' This is perhaps reasonable as they are usually baffled about how to help their partner cope during this intense and challenging experience. It is also often hard for the partners to simply understand the unconscious drive women have to experience childbirth. Gosh, we women don't even understand it!

Having control is very much a part of our value system these days and we feel we must find a way to absolutely ensure we have it. An epidural will, in most cases, ensure you cannot feel the pain. And many women today are saying, 'Well, if it's so painful and so much trouble, why not just have a caesarean and be done with it?' A fair question, but maybe it's a bit like asking, 'If children playing in muddy puddles create so much mess and trouble, why not just control the situation and keep all kids inside?' The reality is that their play is about so much more than getting dirty. It's about learning, creativity, discovery and a preparation for more profound things to come, just as childbirth is. Maybe it's possible, with this in mind, to at least approach childbirth with an attitude of 'giving it a try'.

But, hey, we live in a world of choice, so we can choose to do what we like, particularly when presented with something as challenging as childbirth. Are we, however, making informed and thoroughly researched choices for our childbirths, or is it our fear making the birthing decisions?

If you could learn some simple behavioural tools that will give you incredible control during labour (or at least part of it, knowing that medical backup is still available if you need it or choose it), would you be willing to give it a try? Would you think: 'This sounds interesting; I'd be fascinated to learn more about controlling the pain during labour using my own resources. I can't promise anything right now, but I just might give these methods a try on the day. I can always have the drugs if I need to'? Then...

Our book is for you

Sarah and I spent a year formulating this text to bring the birth skills classes to you. We want, through our text, to come right inside your home where you and your partner will probably be reading this book, so that we can enhance your antenatal education and make sure you both have the skills you need to work as a team during the birth of your child.

Yes, we wrote this book for your partners too. As supportive members of the birth team he (for practical reasons, we refer to your partner as 'he', and the baby as 'she', although we realise this is not always the case) can be inspired by the lessons as well. We want to provide both of you with lessons in self-reliance to better equip you on the day. And this book can be used in conjunction with what you are learning at your hospital or community antenatal classes as they are both valuable, different, compatible and complementary.

Please read the next chapter carefully as it forms the basis of the book. Also pay attention to Sarah's final chapter as it portrays what the rewards of childbirth are really all about. The chapters in between are your skill lessons, which are not complicated, and contain important information for your practice of the skills and further preparation for the birth. You will notice some repetition throughout. This is very much intended. Repetition is intrinsic to labour preparation and recall. Many of my students report back to me that they hear my voice during labour, telling them what to do, and this is because of the repetition. Our aim is for you to remember as much as possible from each chapter so that you are able to recall it when you are in labour and under stress.

Sarah and I will teach you the techniques that regrettably were not available for me when I had my children. They are techniques that Sarah and her husband used so magnificently during the births of their children. I hope you will try them too. I will teach you the individual techniques, explain their physiology and how each one works, and give you the process of how to use each skill, just as I have been instructing the couples in my classes for many years. Sarah will then take you on the same journey of learning that she took as a member of my birth skills classes when she attended during both of her pregnancies. You will be down on the floor with her, learning, laughing and launching into a new set of activities designed to assist you with your contractions. You will become familiar with the techniques from both a teacher's perspective and a learner's experience.

We will also introduce to you many of the other women from classes over the years and this will give you even more ideas about how labour and its pain can be managed in a multitude of ways. You will learn fascinating tools from each person. I never tire of hearing their feedback or reading their stories, and their contributions are a significant and valued part of my classes.

As always with my writing, I like to talk to you as though you are sitting or standing right in front of me in one of my classes. Sarah will talk to you as though you are positioned right next to her during each skills session. So please join us in this series of classes, learning the skills, chapter by chapter, and together let's see if we can change the way you relate to labour pain. Let's see if we can help you with some of the fear you might have, as well. And let's see if we can get you and your partner ready for one of the most incredible adventures of a lifetime.

Your education starts now

I guess the first question you want to ask us is, 'Can you actually master labour pain?' I could answer this for you but it is a question that I want you to answer. However, it is too early for you to do that just yet. It is a question you can address again at the end of the book, after you have learned all the skills. First we have some work to do.

Activity *plus* focus

There is no doubt that labour pain is a perplexing and challenging sensation. It is therefore valuable to work towards solutions that will help you to deal with it, rather than panicking and seeing it only as a problem. A degree of fear, panic and the resulting rise in stress hormones can be useful in labour, but if these three by-products of the pain overwhelm you they will present you with only one option: freezing. This frozen state only compounds the problem, as it creates more fear, more panic, more stress hormones, and ultimately more pain. It makes a solution much more difficult to achieve.

I know it may sound a bit of a cliché, but in childbirth knowledge really is power. In order to master labour pain you need to move from a state of fear, ignorance and anxiety towards focusing on conscious activities to apply to contractions. I specifically use the term 'conscious activities' because you will not only be applying pain-relieving activities to contractions, you will also be concentrating on them. This is an important part of the strategy. Activity *plus* focus. As you learn these skills, your fear will give way to confidence and courage. As you master these simple techniques you will be working towards a richer and more rewarding childbirth experience.

- You will learn what to do with the fear.
- You will learn what to do with the panic.
- You will learn what to do with the stress.
- You will learn what to do with the pain.

In my 30 years of teaching pain mastery techniques for childbirth, I have tried in my classes to integrate the concept of breaking down something that is frightening and seems too hard to deal with, into simple, learnable, achievable parts. It is all about action. Small action. Big action. It is about enlisting activities that align themselves with reducing pain, not increasing it. It is about what works in labour. It is about powerful, realistic resources and human potential. It is about turning ancient gifts into modern skills. It is about empowering you.

Sarah didn't believe these skills would work for her at first. She arrived at my class a little apprehensive ... but I will let her tell you about that.

Sarah's story

I was about six months pregnant with my first child when my obstetrician, Keith Hartman, suggested I take Juju Sundin's birth skills classes. Did I really need to see someone else about my labour? I already planned to take antenatal classes at the hospital I'd booked into for the delivery, The Mater Hospital in Sydney, and I had read countless textbooks about pregnancy and labour. I had seen drawings of a baby in the uterus and pictures of a baby being born. I knew childbirth was incredibly painful. I knew it could take a very long time. And that it is scary. Isn't that all there was to know?

Keith told me that his daughter had taken Juju's classes and that she had had an incredible birth. Now I was intrigued. After reading all those books I certainly didn't feel that I was in for an 'incredible' birth! Then, when I thought about it some more, I realised I didn't actually know what I would be feeling and experiencing once I got into that labour room. What was the pain really like? As far as I knew it was so bad no one liked to talk about it. The books didn't describe it. Women just looked away if I asked; it seemed to be some unspeakable horror. That was it, I decided, I was going to have an epidural. I mean, who gets their teeth pulled without anaesthetic? But Keith persisted. He assured me Juju's classes were unlike any other antenatal class. He was so right.

Juju taught me about the true physiology of pain. By reading this book you will also learn about it – where the pain is, why you feel it, how your mind registers that pain, what your body does during labour, the hormones you will produce and how your baby is born.

I now know that if I hadn't understood all this I wouldn't have lasted very long once my labour pain started. I would have felt scared, unsure and probably would have lost control right away. Juju explained to me how, when you are threatened, there are over a thousand chemical reactions produced in your body. These mobilise the large muscle groups of your body with huge surges of energy so they are ready to help you to attack the situation. If nothing is done when this adrenalin starts pumping the levels will only increase, causing stress and eventually distress and lack of control. Being out of control was certainly not an experience I wanted in my labour.

These are not airy-fairy, hippie, all-natural birthing classes. Juju understands the need for epidurals, for caesareans, for medical intervention. What Juju gives you is the ability to understand your labour so you can make informed decisions throughout about how to cope with the pain. She always says that it doesn't matter how your baby arrives so long as you felt you had some control. We hope these techniques get you the whole way through your labour without intervention but if not we hope you will be inspired by what you can do and in doing so revel in the knowledge that you tried.

This is why I became involved in Juju's book. After my first son was born I thought back to the classes, to my labour and to the excitement, effort and adventure of giving birth to him. When Juju asked if I would be interested in giving a student's perspective in her new book I jumped at the chance. I understood her passion for giving women options by teaching and helping them to dispel their fears of childbirth. I truly believe Juju's birth skills are something every woman should take with her into childbirth.

I feel so lucky I learnt and understood Juju's lessons. I understood what my body was physically doing throughout my labour and when you finish this book you will also have an understanding of the pain of labour, what it is and why you are feeling it. You will be in command of that pain because you are armed with methods that work to help you deal with it.

I hope you find these skills as invaluable as my husband and I have. Giving birth is a miracle. Good luck and enjoy the adventure.

Have you heard the one about instinct and control?

It never surprises me when women from my classes tell me, over and over again, that their instincts did not tell them what to do during their labours. We must recognise that even though our primitive ancestors may have had some very effective instinctive strategies for coping with labour pain, at this point in our history intellectual supremacy and socialisation have overridden them in our consciousness. These instinctive behaviours are still very much there but they just don't seem to come naturally any more. Besides that, our sophisticated consciousness hungers for control over most situations in our lives, so we struggle for the elusive control over labour pain – just expecting it to happen – disappointed and angry when it doesn't.

As I've said, control is a big part of our value system; conversely, we fiercely avoid loss of control. I guess this is related to the rules we have developed as a society, with our emphasis on order rather than chaos. More and more, our ability to tolerate anything that doesn't absolutely suit us seems to be heading south fast. Is it not then unreasonable of us to have the expectation of an instinct suddenly appearing to direct and rescue us in labour and provide us with all the control we are seeking even though women have been having babies for thousands of years?

Instinct is not a commonly used resource in our day-to-day lives, therefore it is a little buried. Try to remember this as you practise the birth skills as they too will not be so familiar to you. But don't worry, most women take a little time to feel comfortable with the skills (Sarah was also a little wary and hesitant at first but was thankful on the day). The aim is to help you to avoid the struggle between your need to have some control over the pain and your fear of losing it.

Healthy pain, healthy responses

During the *first stage* of labour with each contraction of the uterus there is a small amount of dilation (or opening) of the cervix, rotation of the baby and descent of the baby down into the pelvis. In the *second stage* of labour the baby is moving through the birth canal towards your vaginal outlet and then into the outside world. The *third stage*, when the placenta is expelled from the uterus and delivered through the vagina, completes the birthing process. Early in the first stage of labour, as the pain is introducing itself to you, you will be able to manage it using fairly low-key behaviours. If this is during the night, try to go back to sleep or simply lie quietly to conserve your energy. If it is daytime, try to carry on as usual and simply relax during contractions.

At this time you are beginning the important work of closely relating to what your body is doing as it begins the magnificent work of childbirth. If you end up having an extended early phase (sometimes called pre-labour), with contractions starting and stopping or just not progressing, you must conserve as much energy as possible for the hours that lie ahead. For a small number of women it could be a day or two before established labour begins. As labour builds up and the pain increases you will have to quickly analyse the situation and make a decision about what you will do for each contraction. If you decide to continue with the journey and the challenge of childbirth using your own resources, you will be presented with the following choices as each contraction commences:

- 60 seconds of painful helplessness or
- 60 seconds of powerful action.

The first option may make it difficult for you to cope, making labour a real struggle; the other will help you avoid unnecessary pain – and the skills in this book will help you with that second choice.

Labour pain is healthy pain

As labour progresses and the pain really establishes its presence, there will be no time to make decisions about how you will handle each contraction: you will just have to go for it! Your responses will have to be instant with no fear, no inhibition, no uncertainty, no embarrassment. In order for this to be possible, it is essential you understand that labour pain is healthy pain. It is caused by the uterine muscle actually working. It is healthy working pain. That's it! It is not caused by trauma, disease, illness, accident, etc. Even when the pain becomes enormous pain it is still only due to uterine muscle fatigue (called ischaemia). Nothing else. Just muscle tiredness. And because the pain is healthy pain you can be proactive, be powerful, be immersed in your birth skill.

Let me clarify here what 'healthy pain' and 'sick pain' behaviours are. If a pain is sick pain it is natural for you to just curl up and want it to go away and usually get medical help for it. If a pain is healthy pain, you can be proactive and do something about it yourself. More importantly, if any pain is healthy pain but you think it is sick pain, then no matter what you try to do it probably won't work; you will just curl up as though it is sick pain. The downside of not understanding that the pain of labour is a healthy pain is that your 'sick pain' reflexes take over, and your fear/freeze reflex inhibits any form of coping.

A reflex occurs when it is unnecessary for a sensory impulse to reach the brain in order to trigger a response. Instead, the message travels to the spinal cord and a response is triggered. It bypasses your intellectual analysis because it needs to be a fast reaction. A typical reflex is when you quickly pull your hand away from a hot plate on a stove when you didn't realise it was on. It is instantaneous, and is an inherited behaviour rather than a learnt one. You can imagine that if you do not understand the healthy nature of labour pain your fear/freeze reflex will inhibit any form of coping.

Saying to yourself 'healthy pain' like a mantra while in labour will help you really focus on it as a meaningful circumstance, and will help inhibit your brain's unconscious scanner (the amygdala) from sending unhealthy pain alarm bells, which usually results in creating an anxiety state within you – something you want to avoid. The fact that labour pain is healthy pain is the very reason it is possible for you to cope – as long as you know what to do and try to use your intellect as well as your instinctive reflexes. Most women don't understand this (I know Sarah didn't initially).

You can see from the points in 'Natural chemical help' (page 8) that you have so much going for you before you even start labour. Once you blend those physiological facts with the skills you will learn from this book, you have a greater chance of being absorbed in the task of labouring and using everything to your advantage. When you are functioning at your highest possible level during each contraction, your fear and anxiety will be barely detectable. Also, you may be interested to know that at the same time as your body is dealing with pain during birth, all systems and organ functions that provide no immediate contribution to the birth process are depressed or shut down, so that all possible energy can be exclusively reserved for the uterus and your pain-relieving activities.

Don't worry, you won't be alone. Your partner will help you. Your midwife and doctor will support you. Your birthplace will be set up to encourage you to be a healthy human being with healthy human pain.

Natural chemical help

If you have ever wondered about your body's ability to help you during labour, you will never be in doubt again after reading these important facts.

- When a sensation of threat or challenge occurs (such as a spider on your leg, an athlete starting a race, or a painful contraction in labour), over 1,000 chemical reactions are produced within your body and these create dramatic and potentially helpful changes in your behaviour instantly.

- Pain messages travel to your brain via your spinal cord, triggering pain-control impulses from the brain in the form of pain-killing chemicals, endorphins, which act to block further upward painful messages – fewer pain messages means you feel less pain.

- If you create intense competition between pain-free activities and pain, the sophisticated brain will pay attention to the dominance of the pain-free sensations.

- The speed at which pain-dulling messages travel along your nerves to your brain is up to 440 kilometres per hour – just one-hundredth of a second.

- The uptake receptors for endorphins reside in the nerve cells along pain pathways (this was discovered by Dr Candace Pert only in 1973), demonstrating endorphins are related to pain processing.

- Consciously mobilising appropriate skills during times of stress can dull the sensation of pain; that is, simple activities, such as sound and movement during labour, produce even more endorphins.

- If you bombard your nervous system with non-painful thoughts and physical and emotional actions, you can dull your pain further through distraction and redirected focus of attention.

- If you work off your excess adrenalin with sound and activity your oxytocin (a hormone that increases the efficiency of contractions during labour) will flow more proficiently.

- Your endorphin levels rise dramatically in the last trimester of pregnancy in readiness to help you with your labour pain and if you work off your excess stress level (adrenalin) during labour your endorphin levels will increase even more.

Knowledge *is* power

Women no longer learn about labour through observation. We no longer see our mothers, sisters, aunties, cousins or neighbours giving birth, and so we do not see or learn about how women cope with childbirth. Nor do our partners. Education, therefore, plays a vital role in learning how to create helpful responses during contractions. Helpful for your pain, helpful for your labour process, helpful for you and your partner. These responses need to be simple and doable so that the tasks are possible. They also need to make sense. I can assure you that education is not learning unless a connection is made – the 'Oh! I see', or 'I get that now', or 'Yes, now that makes sense'.

If you are frightened of the pain of labour, pat yourself on the back as you are absolutely normal! Human beings have a very strong innate conditioning towards pleasure, but more importantly (also part of our survival reflex) a very powerful pulling away from pain. That is why we panic at the thought of having to face something that we would normally walk away from – too big, too painful, too hard, too frightening! Believe me, I was no different during my births! As well as that, we as women must recognise that we have become very competent in our working and career lives, and yet when we become pregnant we seem to have a big black hole of knowledge regarding labour itself. We have no idea of our capabilities and this is where the fear comes from. So you can see that we have both unconscious and conscious issues that contribute to our fear of childbirth.

Then there are the frightening stories of birth relayed by well-meaning friends and family members. Only this morning, I had a frightened woman on the phone telling me that her girlfriend had told her that labour pain was like the very severe pain of the kidney stones she had passed. Ouch! So already this woman has linked labour pain with sick pain. She was terrified. Fortunately we could talk it through. No one had told her that labour pain is healthy pain. At the beginning of this phone call she was terrified; at the end of it she was empowered.

Labour pain is not like kidney stone pain, or endometriosis pain, or migraine pain, or toothache pain. It is the healthy pain of a muscle working. The uterine muscle working.

Use your skills

Fear is a double-edged sword. Some fear and anxiety in labour can be useful as it will give you the energy and motivation to access helpful behaviours and take control. Excessive fear and panic will lead to distress and the kind of 'frozen' state that leads to helplessness and loss of control, therefore amplifying the very pain you are trying to master. You are going to learn what to do with the fear, the panic, the adrenalin and the pain with the skills in this book.

Coping with labour today is being able to use your intelligence, not just relying on your instinct to just kick in. We will expose you to a rich resource of ideas, knowledge, thoughts, insights, action plans, encouragement and inspiring ways to approach childbirth. You will develop the concept of empowerment that will take you way beyond your day-to-day capabilities. I remember all too well the days of rigid breathing exercises and passive relaxation techniques for labour. I also remember how they zapped women's energy, lengthened their labours and led so quickly to a loss of control. Women frequently said, 'Everything I learned went out the window as soon as I went into labour.' Birth skills will not. They are practical and they are potent.

Does this mean every woman who attends my classes has a drug-free birth? Of course not. There are never any guarantees. Besides that, it's not the aim of birth skills. Maybe you will have a drug-free birth and maybe you won't. No one can possibly know that until the day. Birth skills are about having some control, some command, so that you can look back on the experience and say, 'We did our best and we feel inspired by what we did!'

Childbirth is an intensely personal experience for you and your partner. Although you will both be immersed in it when it happens, it is only you, the woman, who will feel the physical pain (your partner may feel it on an emotional level, though). That is why the major learning impact needs to be on you – your skills, your knowledge, your wisdom, your ability. This focus on you, the woman learning the skills, in no way diminishes the role of your partner. Actually it enhances it, as each of you will understand exactly what your individual roles are. As you continue with your learning, try to make sense of what birth skills are all about. Rather than having a black hole of awareness, these skills are about understanding what is going on in the inner world of your labouring body.

Birth skills are about managing the pain sensation that accompanies each contraction and also about managing yourself: after all, the pain doesn't mind if you lose control – only you do! You need to accept that with contractions there will be some pain, but only a small part of you will actually be in pain each time a contraction comes (the low to mid abdomen, or the low back or the outside of the thighs during the first stage of labour; in the second stage of labour primarily in the vaginal outlet as the baby crowns). The rest of you is pain free! When you go into labour, you will know how to recruit some or all of these pain-free parts of yourself to help you manage the part of you that is in pain. Let's be more specific. Your head is not in pain, nor are your eyes, your ears, your nose, mouth, lungs, hands, back, chest, legs, nor your feet, nor most of the skin on your body. You are going to use all these pain-free parts to help you manage the small part of your body that will be in pain.

For most women in most labours, only the contraction part has pain: the time in between will be pain free. So, for example, in a 12-hour labour, perhaps only a total of four contraction hours of it will have really challenging pain. Maybe less. We tend to 'forget' about the pain-free periods in between the contractions. These are an important part of labour and you will use them to do nothing except rest until the next contraction.

Here is something else to ponder before you go any further. It is something I mention in class all the time:

We all have the potential to experience unbelievable pain in labour, but we also have the potential to produce behaviours and actions that can reduce it.

This needs to be part of your belief system. I am going to remind you yet again: your physiology is 'for you', not 'against you'.

And finally ...

If you think labour is only about having a baby and enduring pain, then you are wrong. Labour is about having a baby, it is about having pain, but is also about that rite of passage in which you have the opportunity to mobilise your skills in order to be in command of something that might otherwise seem too big to handle. This is what most women approaching childbirth do not know. Sarah's final chapter, 'The bigger picture', will help you to fully comprehend this. There is no doubt that a sense of mastery during the experience of childbirth can offset the negative aspects of the stress.

You will have to accept that you have no direct control over the contractions or the level of pain, so don't waste time on trying to control what you can't; instead put 120 per cent of your energy into what you can control. You absolutely can have control over:

- what you do with your legs and hands
- what you do with your breath and sound
- what you do with your eyes and ears
- what you do with your nose and skin
- what you do with your thoughts and words
- how you use the muscles needed to push out your baby.

This is what birth skills are all about. You will learn how to reshape some of your behaviours, the ones you do have control over, the ones that are entirely appropriate for labour pain management, so that you can, with your partner, and your astounding capabilities, master your own pain. Never underestimate your own power.

Your first skill in mastering labour pain is 'Movement'.

Skills for the *first stage* of labour

Movement

The day I gave birth to my daughter Heidi started like any other day. I was two weeks overdue and by two or three o'clock that afternoon it was clear to me that the backache I was experiencing was actually labour. This was a long time ago: 14 July 1980, wintertime in Australia. I spent the next 12 hours at home coping with the increasingly painful contractions by simply walking, sitting, breathing (and complaining, as I recall!), standing and swaying in front of the heater (it was a cold winter that year), leaning over the kitchen bench, showering, lying down for a rest then, as the next contraction came, getting up from the couch and pacing again and so on. All this seemed quite normal to me and the appropriate thing to do when one was in pain.

The trip to the hospital was swift, thankfully, and after an initial examination I was taken to my room. Then, for the next eight hours – that is, for the duration of the rest of my labour – I lay on a bed, on my back, in agony, as my husband sat on a chair beside me.

In the good ol' days

My labour had changed from being reasonably tolerable at home and in the car, to becoming absolutely unbearable the moment I lay on that bed in the delivery suite. The pain was increasing and I needed to do something! Anything! But no, it was not the way things were done. I did not understand why I was restricted to the bed, yet I accepted it – that's what everyone did. It was perplexing and frustrating that I was able to do as I wished during the pain of the first part of the labour while I was at home, but now I was not free to do as I wished to try to manage the most enormous pain I had ever had in my life. I had to stay passive, in a reclining position, when all I wanted to do was to continue what I was doing at home, perhaps with some extra tools later on as the pain increased and the contractions accelerated.

If you ask your own mothers about their births, I'm sure many will have a similar story. For me that was over a quarter of a century ago and it is a reflection of the social sets of rules in delivery suites at the time. There was no particular reason for the positional and movement or behavioural limitations other than that it was normal for people to lie down in hospitals. No one questioned it. Everyone just did it and certainly no one was to be blamed. I'm positive it was right there, on that bed, that I formulated what I would be doing in my career as a physiotherapist for many, many years to come.

Restricted to a bed? It just didn't make sense! Not being able to continue what was working so well at home? Crazy! The same legs that took me up and down my hallway at my house, stepped up and down on the spot in front of the heater in my family room, felt the cold soothing sensation of the tiles on the kitchen floor for a change of feeling on the soles of my feet, now detached and lifeless on the bed. Looking back now, I just shake my head and wonder why I didn't question it. Well, social sets of rules evolve and are meant to be broken. I then spent the next 25 years contributing to that evolution.

FELICITY *I used the sound of my bare feet slapping on the bathroom floor. I was really focused on the sound and the sensation of this. Later I used the deep bath and made similar splashing noises with my feet on the side of the bath. This was essential for focusing and I dilated from 6 to 10 centimetres in 15 minutes. Amazing!*

Fast-forward ...

Today, unless there is a medical reason the mother needs to be restricted to the bed in labour, every woman is able to choose what she does. If the bed is where she wants to be, then that is one of her options; if that's not where she wants to be, no problem. The point is, the labouring woman can stand, sit, lie down, kneel, lean, walk or find any position that suits her. Delivery suites in hospitals are warm and welcoming and are set up for total freedom so you have the choice to do whatever you need to in order to manage your labour.

HEATHER *On admission, I began rhythmically and lightly stomping around the room. I liked the feel and sound of my feet on the linoleum floor. As the pain built I progressed to heavier stomping. Fatigue caught up with me and I sat on the fit ball and tapped my heels on the floor. This progressed to massive pounding of my feet on to the vinyl floor mattress. Eventually I changed my breathing to a very loud 'Aahh' sound and all of this got me to 10 centimetres.*

Legs for labour

This is a special class in my programme in which women are taught all the different ways they can use their legs (and their hips and feet) to help master contraction pain and to facilitate the labour process. It is one of my favourite classes because it is so simple and at the end of it the women say to me, 'Wow! I didn't know I could do this!' Actually, it's one of the 'Now I get it' classes – every teacher's dream.

I first conducted 'Legs for Labour' the week after attending the world-famous soprano, Joan Sutherland's, final performance at the Sydney Opera House in October 1990. You might be wondering what connection I made between singing and leg activity for labour pain. I didn't! The connection came *after* the singing! Once the applause began, I found myself right inside one of the most incredibly powerful and uplifting experiences you could ever imagine. You really could say 'the house came down'!

As 'La Stupenda' stood graciously on the stage in the most amazing dress to take her final bow, hundreds of people (1,600 to be exact) rose to their feet and clapped and yelled and stamped. And stamped harder, and louder, and harder again. And clapped faster, and yelled even louder. I guess there were some 'Bravos' in there somewhere but the noise was so loud it was impossible to discern them. Thousands of beautiful daffodils hurtled towards the stage from members of the audience; hundreds and hundreds, probably thousands, of streamers were tossed from every corner in the hope of reaching the stage. And the stamping continued, louder, harder, faster, and then the fireworks began. The cast and the members of the orchestra, who had gathered around her onstage, joined in. They had their own turn at stamping, frenzied stamping, and then the audience started again, stamping, stamping louder, more streamers, more daffodils, then a deafening sound from the cast onstage, then the audience again in response, and more fireworks. I seriously began to doubt the floor could support it all!

This expression of joy and appreciation and farewell to a great artist continued for 20 to 30 minutes, until all that was left was the smell of the smoke from the burnt-out fireworks and an almost reluctant curtain coming down for the final time. As I slumped exhausted yet exhilarated in my seat I realised the value of using the legs for expression. Any expression. Not just for joy and exuberance as in the Sydney Opera House, but for the expression of pain in labour. And especially for turning fear and pain into positive action by harnessing the adrenalin in our bodies and turning it into action. I was damn sure the women in my classes could do this during labour. So my 'Legs for Labour' class came into being.

What does it involve? Well, we examine leg movements for expressions of pain, for distraction, for endorphin mobilisation, as a primary tool, as a secondary tool, to use with counting and visualisation, while in the shower or the bath, or on the fit ball. So you can see there is so much more to do than just walk around in labour.

ALICIA *Of all the techniques I learned, my legs felt the most natural. In the delivery room, I was encouraged by my midwife to pace the floor, breathe deeply and remain calm. When the contractions intensified I stood at the foot of the bed for support and stomped on the spot. My shoes made a loud clatter on the wooden floor. I used this sound for distraction. I increased the speed and the sound before the peak of the contraction to best distract my mind from the pain. When I tired from being in an upright position I knelt face down into a bean bag and kicked my legs on the soft floor mattress. I used this kicking right up until the pushing phase. Adapting to the pain with my legs was for me a very effective resource for mastering labour pain.*

A little physiology ...

In any threat or crisis in our lives – and dealing with labour pain is one of those times – our fight or flight reflex kicks in. An instant rush of adrenalin, that fantastic hormone of action, brings about major changes, resulting in what is called the 'general adaptation syndrome'. This is the mechanism through which we can quickly adapt in order to manage the threat or crisis at hand, particularly if it is dangerous or life threatening or overwhelming.

Childbirth is not dangerous but most would agree it is overwhelming in the sense that the pain of the contractions changes from the level of mild period pain to the greatest pain most of us will ever feel. The physiological and psychological detail of the fight or flight response is complex but it is important to understand that our large muscle groups – the largest being our legs – undergo instant surges of energy during times of need so they may be recruited to help us to immediately adapt to the crisis situation. This means we are given physiological capabilities to use our legs to help us cope with the pain and not lose control.

Think for a moment about some of the many possibilities of threat or crisis that may need instant and enormous surges of energy:

- to climb a tree to get away from an angry dog – hurry!
- to jump and run to escape a sudden big wave on the beach – quick!
- to kick at a predator to protect yourself – get away!
- to yell loudly for assistance – H E L P!

I have used these examples as they are fast response incidences but we all know that stress can also be caused by thousands, millions, of other things that have a slower, more agitating effect, such as loud, irritating music, a faulty exhaust on a car, an unpleasant smell, slow traffic, fast traffic, work problems, a moth buzzing around the ceiling at night and even irritating static in your telephone. Only the other day I was at the supermarket and as usual I was in a hurry. When I finally got near the front of the queue the customer ahead of me began a long conversation about rising costs! Silly, I know, but I began to feel a low-grade churning stress. It's happened to all of us. However, it is the instant response-type stress I want you to think about here – the fast stuff!

The sensations of early contractions in labour are a little like the slower, more agitating stress, and you will probably find you don't need anything in particular to help you cope – some will, but most of you won't. But these early contractions usually don't cause a crisis. Established labour pain, especially when it gets more and more intense, moves from being mildly agitating to eventually bringing about a crisis situation in your body, even though the pain is healthy pain. So let's talk about this concept of healthy pain a bit more.

It's a muscle at work

A contraction of the uterus in labour is no different to a contraction of any muscle used in a challenging gym workout, during which you are using your muscles in a healthy way. Is a gym workout pain free? Nope! In fact it's the painful contractions that actually strengthen your muscles (as it is the painful contractions in labour that really do the work).

Labour pain comes from muscle fatigue (just as in a gym workout) as your uterus contracts and relaxes repetitively over the hours of labour.

If childbirth comprised only one hour of contractions, then none of us would ever experience the level of pain we do; the uterine muscle would not have time to tire. When any muscle in the body gets tired it sends out a pain signal via the nervous system. These types of muscle contractions are similar to the pain you feel from your abdominals or your hamstrings or your biceps or your quadriceps if you exercise them for long enough. Healthy activities create healthy, workable forms of pain.

Now, if you have a personal trainer to help you exercise you can do it for a lot longer than you might if you exercised alone! This is because when any sort of pain takes you out of your comfort zone you want to stop. But a coach can keep you going, and usually with very simple techniques. It might be something as simple as them saying, 'Just one more, you can do it, just one more!' One of the couples (Deb and Pete) from my classes adopted this exact mantra and used it successfully all the way through the labour (read Deb's excerpt in Skill # 5). So you see, labour pain is quite a simple pain: it's only the pain of a muscle contracting. And in labour, your partner can be your coach.

So how can the fight/flight reflex help you and why on earth would the legs need a surge of adrenalin in labour when all you are doing is having a baby?

CHLOE *You [Juju] were right. You can't stay still during the intense pain. I stamped my feet and pretended I was power walking, which I had done for years. I focused on the sound of the clonk, clonk, clonk noise my trainers made on the floor. I was counting and stomping throughout every contraction. It all made such sense. My use of breath and, later, the 'Aahh' sound with the stomp stopped me from tensing up.*

Leg work is pain free

Using your legs is one way to adapt easily to the stress of labour and to take control of your contraction pain. Leg activity changes your perception of pain by stimulating sensations at the sensory receptor sites, which are in the soles of your feet, the skin on your legs, receptors in your hips and knees and ankles, etc. These sensations, which are pain-free sensations, are then transferred to the brain. If you generate enough leg activity, your brain will register this pain-free leg activity rather than the uterine pain, as the brain can only focus on one thing at a time and it will always focus on the dominant sensation. This concept will apply to each skill you learn in this book, not just the legs. Essentially, you will override the painful sensations by bombarding your brain with sensations that are pain free. You will be making the pain-free activity the dominant sensation because:

- your legs provide a natural and familiar activity to focus on rather than concentrating on the pain
- leg activity is naturally rhythmic and this rhythm is fundamental to focusing
- you can easily use other techniques, such as counting and breathing, in time with your steps and movements, increasing the impact of your pain-control repertoire
- constant leg activity will help you work off your adrenalin, so the levels don't get too high and work against you and your labour, possibly causing more pain and stress
- leg work will help you increase your endorphin levels (in the same way a gym workout does) therefore helping to neuro-chemically block your pain.

The inside job

When labour begins, the pain is mostly mild to moderate. Most women, but not all, manage this early pain of the first stage of labour with gentle, passive activities, such as relaxation techniques, breathing awareness, a warm bath or heat pack, calming music, or even simply lying down and trying to go back to sleep. The contractions may only last for 15 to 20 seconds with a long break between each one but things are starting to move inside.

If you could look inside your body at this point, you would see your cervix (the lower part of the uterus) starting to efface, meaning the cervix, which has been tightly closed for nine months, is thinning and pulling upwards to be incorporated with the lower part of the uterus. You cannot actually feel your cervix effacing but the contractions will proceed to open the cervix over several hours to about 10 centimetres. It is good to have strong images in your mind of the diameters of dilation. The diagram below shows you the size at 1, 3, 5, 8 and 10 centimetres. The contractions also exert some turning pressure on the baby and move the baby deeper into your pelvis ready for the pushing phase. You cannot feel these internal activities of dilation, rotation or descent but you will feel the muscle fatigue that results from the uterus making these activities happen.

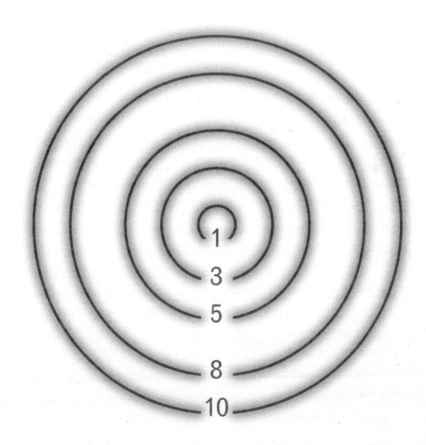

In a nutshell, you will feel the power and the pain from the contractions, but not the birthing activities occurring inside your body. This is one of the things that makes childbirth difficult, but the skills in this book will help you to adjust to the pain. Mild pain requires mild adaptation, moderate pain requires moderate adaptation, big pain requires big adaptation, and so on. There is no specific recipe for the right time to use a particular skill. Try them all at different times. Find out which one works best for you.

Then what happens

The pain, for most women, runs in a band about the size of a sports sock across the low abdomen or the low back or sometimes the thighs. It is usually in only one of these places at any one time. If it gets out of control, though, it can feel like it is everywhere, even in your toes! In the first stage of labour, as the cervix continues to open and the baby moves deeper into the pelvis, the pain naturally increases as the contraction work increases. For most women, the pain occurs only during contractions; the rest of the time they are pain free. As labour becomes established and the pain starts to take you out of your comfort zone, the length of the contractions will usually be around 60 seconds. The intervals in between will vary, but these intervals will get shorter. It is the 60-second periods of pain that we are most interested in with pain mastery. During the in-between periods you will be resting. And that means doing nothing, just resting!

When the pain increases even more in intensity during the 60-second contractions, it creates more stress, so the body accordingly produces more adrenalin to provide you with the potential for more energy and therefore more appropriate pain-reducing adaptation – that is, a faster pace with the feet stomping rather than slow pacing, vocalising rather than breathing. Research has shown that the level to which women master their labour pain depends on two things:

1. the level of pain
2. their ability to adapt.

You cannot change the level of pain but you can adapt so that you indirectly lower your feeling of that level of pain! I guess we could call pain mastery, pain adaptability. It's exactly the same thing, but it will build up to be massive adaptability. Whatever techniques you use.

Contraction pain involves exposing you to small manageable amounts of stress that increase as the labour progresses (remember it's only a muscle working! The uterine muscle working! The uterine muscle tiring! Healthy work, healthy pain!) Unless you gradually adapt to these increasing amounts of stress they will become unmanageable. In the labour context 'adapting' means applying activity to these 60-second periods of pain. It can be active or passive, mental or physical, or a mix.

Note the repetition – I did warn you! But it really does make for solid learning.

VERONICA *Throughout my four labours I used many techniques to cope with pain but there was one I used through them all: I walked and walked and walked during the contractions. I sat down between each one. When I was too tired to walk I lay on the bed and maintained leg motion as though I was walking. It was sort of like pedalling a bike as I lay on my side. Sometimes I would just rub my feet together. My body made me do it. I couldn't stop it and I didn't want to. If I couldn't have done it, I wouldn't have coped.*

Let's talk about adrenalin

Adrenalin 'thinks' in terms of stress and action. If action is not taken when adrenalin pumps into your system – even if the trigger is healthy pain – it will continue to rise and rise within your body, increasing your stress. If you don't adapt to it, your rising stress may become distress – a state everyone wants to avoid. This invariably leads to panic and loss of control. If you can mobilise yourself with a pain-free rhythmic activity (think '*legs, legs, legs*'!) and focus on that, believe me, fear and panic will take a back seat. If you do something and focus on it, you will have a decreased conscious ability to register fear and panic, and you will definitely decrease your brain's perception of the pain. *Remember:* During a contraction, pain produces stress, which triggers the adrenalin pump that fuels the action you need to take in order to cope.

If your adrenalin could talk during contractions it would say, 'Come on, do something!' Unfortunately, it is one of the few hormones in the body that cannot naturally deplete itself. It has to have activity of some kind to release it and burn it up to prevent you building up into a state of distress. Pain mastery involves working off this stress while it surges into your body as the painful contractions build up. If you panic and freeze and 'hang on' to your adrenalin the result will be:

- more pain as high adrenalin levels negatively affect your tension and endorphin release
- a less efficient labour as high adrenalin levels negatively affect oxytocin released to your brain.

If this continues, you will find it enormously difficult to maintain any command or control over your labour.

Adrenalin, in high levels with the really heavy pain, is there for a purpose. Usually we, as human beings, solve most of our problems with thinking skills but this may not be appropriate for established labour. The adrenalin rush is designed to make you bypass your own thinking and create instant action. You see, when the pain builds to enormous levels, thinking about what to do with it may take too long and will result in you feeling the full force of the pain, especially in transition as you dilate from about 7 to 10 centimetres in the first stage of labour. When the big ones start coming you need instant action. This is exactly what adrenalin does for you. It doesn't want you to relax. It wants you to 'Go'!

Think of an athlete starting a race. The alert/priming for action phase is created for him when the marshal says, 'On your mark,' and it is further enhanced with the 'Get set' – both of these processes last no longer than two to three seconds. Then the 'Go' message is sent. We don't need a marshal during labour; our body with its general adaptation reflexes does that for us. Just make sure you don't stay in the 'On your mark' and 'Get set' phases for the whole contraction; spend most of the painful contractions in the 'Go' phase. Imagine if that same marshal said, 'On your mark ... Get set ... Relax,' or 'On your mark ... Get set ... Freeze'! The athlete would miss the race. There could be no race. Your contraction may not be a race, but you still have the same sequence of fight/flight physiology happening. 'Go' (as opposed to 'Relax') is a great keyword for your partner to use if you are having trouble getting out of the shock/freeze state. Too many couples persist with 'Relax', when it is obvious the woman is way past achieving this. Move on to the 'Go' words and activities.

Many women freeze in response to the energy rush in well-established labour because they don't understand it. It is powerful – Sarah describes her body in labour as 'bursting with energy' – and it can shock you rather than help you. Don't be frightened by it. All that is happening is that the alerting, priming part of the rush is so big and so sudden it may cause you to extend the two-to-three-second 'wake up' phase of it for the duration of the contraction, rather than motivating you to action.

Repetition! It's part of the process. Read the previous paragraph again. I want you to be fascinated by your own body chemistry, not fearful of it. I want you to understand it on the deepest possible level. And respect it. This is why I go over and over and over the physiology of childbirth in my classes, and why I am doing the same in this book.

Try to see the existence of adrenalin as an incredible advantage, a chemical that gives you much greater speed and ability to react than you could ever muster up without it. Try to work with it, allow it to do what it is designed to do to help you when you need it in labour – an instant action, not too big, not too small, but just right to match the pain.

ANNA *Having spent years horse riding, it seemed only natural to combine a rhythmic sitting/bouncing/rocking action on the fit ball, which I used like a saddle, holding on to the metal bar at the foot of the delivery bed as the reins. I visualised myself riding through the contractions as my husband kept breathing with me throughout the 60-second duration. This worked brilliantly to block the pain.*

Labour is not easy

You will hear the 'match the pain' statement many times throughout this book. In labour you are presented with incredible pain to deal with, but make no mistake, you are also programmed and equipped with a series of reflex adaptations that kick into gear when the pain starts. If you know what to do, and if you put hesitation and inhibition on the back burner for a few hours, for each 60-second duration of pain, you can apply, instantly, the resources required to see you through. You may indeed use a 'mix' of resources to increase your adaptation as the pain requires, but the programming to do this is already in place.

The bottom line is, the pain (the stress) produces the mechanism (adrenalin surge) to protect you (creating your ability to adapt quickly) from the pain (by blocking it). The more you explore and focus on your non-painful skills, the less you will feel any fear – remember, the brain can focus only on one thing at a time. If you are in a 'flow', or 'zone', with your skills, you will suspend fear, inhibition, panic and hesitation. You must focus on the non-painful activity for this to work well. Use whatever you need. If you are using leg work and it helps you more to count out aloud in time to your steps, then do it. If it helps you more to listen to your partner or extra support people doing this, then do that. If it helps to watch your partner do it, then do that too – everyone can be involved. You will not be alone but very much part of a team.

Remember adrenalin: what would it say? '*Come on, do something!*' This chemical would not be there if we were meant to be passive during contractions.

Once you understand this physiology you will never have to read it again. I never teach anything in my classes without explaining the 'why' of everything. Make sure your partner knows it too as it will help him understand what this is all about. As well as being the support person and coach, he may also need to be the marshal sometimes. The physiology here applies to all the chapters that follow, so keep it fresh in your mind.

KIELY *I began using my legs at home even though the pain was not too intense at this stage. I just needed to get my mind off it. I focused on the movements of my legs and counting the taps I made with them against a door. Why I did this I do not know. It just happened. When it came time to go to the hospital I wanted to take that door with me! In the car I marched my feet to the rhythm of the tune on the car radio. I also began banging stress balls together. I was 10 centimetres on admission. During pregnancy I had been terrified of childbirth – and I mean terrified! Using my legs meant that I mastered the pain and felt in control. I was amazed I could do this!*

There was a time ...

Sometimes the women in my class bring their mothers along to see what their daughters are learning. I love these classes because before us we have three generations: the soon-to-be grandmother, the soon-to-be mother and the child (in utero). The night Sarah brought her mother the topic was Legs for Labour. It was incredible to see another woman from my own generation listen so intently and take part in all the practical work with great enthusiasm and without one moment of hesitation. When I talked to her after the class and asked her about this she said: 'I had nothing like this when I had my children, it's brilliant, and it all makes so much sense!' Sarah's mum also added, 'Compared to how it was for us, these women don't know how lucky they are.'

Women of our generation learned either nothing or the psychoprophylaxis (not a user-friendly label) method for their births. Our generation really did struggle on those beds. It wasn't like that for every-one, nothing ever is, but most of us had a really hard time getting through labour. I would like you to answer this question: Would you rather give birth restricted to a bed, not being able to use your legs as you are so cleverly programmed to do, or give birth with the freedom to do whatever it takes to deal with the pain?

If you choose freedom, then when those painful contractions come, *put your legs to work*, make them *work harder* than the pain, and *focus on your legs*, not the pain.

Movement skills

Practise these skills during pregnancy so they are second nature when you go into labour. Add your own variations at any time and read the excerpts from members of my classes (scattered throughout this chapter and at the end) to get more ideas for leg activities. Practise those as well. They provide many insights about labour and many ideas about how to use your legs to master contraction pain in the first stage of labour. There is no particular order or mix when applying the behaviours during labour: do whatever feels right for you at the time.

ROCK AND SWAY

As you stand, rock and sway rhythmically from side to side. Feel your body and the baby's weight exerting gentle sideways pressure over each of your legs and feet as you move. Focus on this. Try to breathe in and out, timing each breath with your movement. Place your hands over your abdomen; perhaps try holding a heat pack over the area of pain.

Add another step: Lean over on to a support and have your partner hold a hot pack over your back or a cool pack over your neck. **Focus on your legs, not the pain.**

PACING THE FLOOR

Pace the floor in a slow, rhythmic fashion while you massage your abdomen at the same time. Breathe slowly in time with your pacing, reminding yourself that everything is happening as it should.

Add another step: Count your steps as you pace up and down the room, hallway, hospital foyer, courtyard, etc. **Focus on your legs, not the pain.**

RHYTHMIC STEPPING

Walk on the spot, focusing on the rhythm of your steps. Count or breathe rhythmically in time with your legs. Feel the floorboards, carpet, soft floor mattress, cold tiles, etc., under your feet. Try this with bare feet, warm socks, trainers.

Add another step: Picture the inside of your body, visualising your cervix opening. Then focus outside of your body, maybe concentrating on a spot on the wall. Increase your pace and breath, as you wish.

Add another step: Say the mantra, 'Keep moving. Keep moving. Keep moving.' Say it out loud.

Accelerate your walking to a harder stomp if the pain increases and takes your attention. **Focus on your legs, not the pain.**

FLOOR MAT MARCHING

Position yourself on all fours, perhaps on the large vinyl floor mattress used during labour. Kick your feet up and down onto one or two pillows placed under them. Increase the kick as your pain increases – faster, harder.

Note: Many women, who prefer this hands and knees position, say they cannot move around much. Actually, you can still move. You can easily and effectively use foot movements, hip rocking, hip swaying, hip rolling, even rocking your whole body backwards and forwards and the movement's momentum makes up for the gravity you would have had if you were upright. Try it now, practise it, and it will become second nature when you need it on the day.

Add another step: Use one hand or a stress ball to tap rhythmically on the floor or on another support.

Note: This is a great position for a backache labour. **Focus on your feet (or hands), not the pain.**

WATER STOMPING

In the shower, stomp your feet and feel the splash under them. Listen to it. Increase your stomping as you need to, to master the pain.

Add another step: Add a few drops of lime or grapefruit oil to the floor of the shower and allow the steam to bring the aroma to your nose for extra distraction. Visualise the fruits.

Add another step: Add an 'Aahh' sound; say it over and over. Grab the metal bar for support.

Add another step: If you are reclining in a bath, tap your feet rhythmically on the enamel and feel the pressure of the spa jets, if your bath has these, on your thighs. **Focus on your feet, not the pain.**

CALF SLIDING

Lying on your side on the bed or on a floor mattress, slide your upper foot along the calf of your lower leg – you can add powder or oil to your leg to enhance the sliding action or just use the natural slide your skin provides. Breathe in time with the slide. If your sliding leg tires, lie on your other side and use the alternative leg.

Add another step: Upbeat music may help with rhythm, and slow music with relaxation (use earphones and an MP3 player rather than a general sound system, to bring the music inside you). Try it in the bath as well.

Note: This is a great position and activity for distraction with a backache labour. **Focus on your feet, not the pain.**

WALL SLIDING

Stand with your back against a wall and use your leg muscles to slide or jiggle your back up and down the wall. Use a rhythm that gives you the sensation of jiggling or sliding away the pain. This could be a slow movement or a faster jiggle or somewhere in between. You could try this against the side of a deep warm spa, if you have one, jiggling up and down in the water, in the squat position.

Add another step: Slide/rock sideways against the wall.

Add another step: Use vocalisation, aromatherapy, keywords or visualisations to help maintain rhythm and enhance distraction. **Focus on your legs, not the pain.**

PALMS ON THIGHS

Kneel on a floor mattress and place one or two pillows between your heels and your buttocks, so there is no pressure on your lower legs as you sit back on them. Rub your palms rhythmically along the outsides of your thighs and count in your head (or out loud) in time with the movements. Incorporate the 'Aahh' sound when the pain builds up. Do the same rubbing on the fronts of your thighs.

Add another step: Pat your thighs lightly and rhythmically with your open palms and notice the pressure and the sound on your thighs. You can increase this as you require – faster, harder – and alternate with the rubbing as it uses different muscles in your arms if they tire.

Note: Your partner can place a citrus-scented tissue under your nose every 15 seconds for extra distraction.

Be aware of the sensation you create between your palms and your thighs. **Focus on your thighs, not the pain.**

FIT BALL BOUNCE

Sit on the ball, supporting yourself well with your feet wide apart. Bounce softly, lifting your heels up and down on the floor in the same rhythm as the bounce. At any time and as you need it, add sounds, smells, imagery, heat and visualisations and concentrate on the rhythm. *Note*: Place a towel over the fit ball, especially if your membranes are leaking. **Focus on your feet, not the pain.**

Cautions

- Wear your trainers if they are more comfortable, especially if you are on your feet for a long time.
- Wear socks if your feet are cold but be careful not to slip in them.
- Be careful not to trip on mats, leads or cords as you move about.
- If your shower is in a bathtub you must support yourself on handrails.
- Make sure there is a non-slip bath mat to move on.
- When using the fit ball be sure to steady yourself against a table, bed, window sill, sink, chair, shower rail or your partner so it doesn't roll from underneath you.
- If your legs tire quickly or if you have swollen legs or varicose veins, or pre-existing leg trauma or injury, monitor the use of your legs carefully and check your movements with your doctor.

Partner's role

- Don't let her start these skills too early in labour as she may tire.
- Check her choice of footwear – shoes, socks, bare feet – to make sure she is comfortable.
- Have your equipment ready: a plastic chair or stool for the shower, tissues for oil (check her fragrance preferences), fit ball, etc.
- Count her into the contraction: 'It's starting in three seconds, get ready, start now!' – use a stopwatch if it helps keep track.
- Pace and walk and step with her.
- Encourage her to move in rhythm with her breathing.

- Count as she paces, in rhythm.

- Stomp with her if necessary.

- Keep her focused on her feet.

- Repeat keywords (see Skill # 5) as she moves.

- Play rhythmic music according to her preferences.

- Apply hot packs to her pain as she requires it.

- Apply cool packs to her forehead.

- Do not encourage a movement that does not come naturally to her.

- Keep her focused on the action and don't talk about other things during the 60-second period of pain.

- Help her to rest between contractions or change strategy if she tires during a skill.

- Give her all the encouragement you can!

A story to encourage you

Do you remember the incredible story of medical student Roger Bannister, who, in 1954, was the first man to run a mile in less than four minutes? Of this experience, he said:

> *For the last 59 seconds there was no pain, only a great unity of movement and aim. The world seemed to stand still or did not exist. The only reality was the next 200 yards of track under my feet. I had a moment of mixed joy and anguish when my mind took over. It raced well ahead of my body and drew my body compellingly forward. I was feeling so tremendously full of running my legs seemed to meet no resistance at all, as if propelled by some unknown force. I was relaxed, so much so, that my mind seemed almost detached from my body ...*

Wow! How motivating! How inspirational! Roger Bannister broke the record and was an incredible role model for runners of his generation and later ones. He felt it was his mental limitations that needed to be broken through to reach his full potential. When you are in labour:

- Is there more that you can do to push through your mental barriers?
- Do you want to discover your incredible potential?
- Can you focus on the 'track' beneath your feet and chant, 'Keep moving,' for 59 seconds of each contraction?

You can certainly have a darn good try! Remember, there is tremendous reward in just trying.

After the birth of her first child, Sarah told me something I will always remember about her and her husband's method:

If he moved, I went too, and if I moved he came with me. We were never alone, we were such a team.

This, for two people in a stressful situation, is movement in the deepest sense.

Sarah's story

The movement class was my first class with Juju. Before I arrived I expected to be just sitting in a chair and being lectured to about the mechanics of labour and birth. Instead I found myself in a large room filled with very pregnant women clustered around, relaxing, chatting and laughing.

Juju welcomed each student individually, by name. The atmosphere was of excitement and anticipation. I didn't know why. I didn't even know the topic of the class as I had started in the middle of the term! I was the newcomer and I felt like it was the first day of school. So I found a nice corner to sit in to make myself inconspicuous ... okay I had a huge belly but, hey, so did everyone else! But I was ready to learn.

Because Juju is a physiotherapist her classes are focused on practicality. She got us up and standing and moved us all into the centre of the classroom. I was uncomfortable; I wanted to hide away in my corner. Juju instructed us to get moving and to think of marching, pacing, stepping or walking on the spot. The other women stood with their feet shoulder-width apart and started stomping their feet up and down. I was taken aback. 'How embarrassing,' I thought. 'And what does this have to do with labour?' I wondered.

I started tiptoeing. Little movements. Looking around to see if anyone was watching. They weren't. Some had their eyes closed and were counting. Others were looking at the floor in concentration. No one cared what anyone else was doing, it was their labour, their experience, their class. I could see all these women empowering themselves, preparing themselves for what was to come. I reluctantly began moving a little bit more to see if I could feel the same way.

As we stomped our feet, Juju led us into making long 'Aahh' sounds in time with our movements. This sounds weird, right? I remember thinking, 'What does this have to do with managing labour pain?' If only I had known then what I know now.

Many women, including me, use movement to master their labour pain. Let me give you an example of a Juju exercise to demonstrate the reasoning behind this. She asked us to stand with our arms outstretched, parallel to the floor. She wanted us to build a form of healthy pain for us to practise with to prepare us for working with labour pain. As we can't practise with our actual uterus, of course, Juju uses our arms to make a muscle work until it is painful. We stood still and twisted the full length of our arms back and forth, keeping them at 90 degrees, for a long time. A very long time.

Granted, our arms have smaller muscles compared with the uterine muscle but the pain was still awful. Faces were scrunching up in agony. Is this nearly over, everyone was thinking. I'd had it. Moaning noises were becoming louder. Arms were drooping. But Juju has eyes in the back of her head and she notices if you slack off and tells you to straighten your arms out again and keep going! She would say, 'Isn't the pain awful? Don't you want it to stop?' 'Yes,' everyone groaned. 'We've had enough. Make it stop! And give us a reason for having to endure this awful exercise!'

In order to increase our tolerance of the pain Juju said we must get bigger than the pain. So for the next part she asked us to keep our arms going but to now also stomp our feet: one, two; one, two. 'Focus on the feet,' she said.

Wow! The arm pain was easing. I hardly noticed it now. The awful pain was still there but as long as I moved my feet and focused on them, I could hardly feel it in my arms. 'A-ha!' The penny dropped.

This exercise showed us just how awful labour pain would be if we froze and did nothing. But the real test was when we stopped moving our feet and kept our arms going. Ouch! We were back to the awful pain again, with nothing to distract us. This was when I became a believer.

KATHRYN *Due to my baby being posterior, one of the most comfortable positions for me was lying on my side and rubbing my feet together. With each contraction I would rub the arch of my upper foot against the inside of my lower foot, which was stationary. I did this in rhythm with each breath out and hit the stress ball against the bed. My mind was focused on my feet and as the contractions intensified the firmness of my foot movements increased, to a point of a mild burning sensation on the inside of my feet.*

You can truly manage pain if you bombard your senses with alternative activities and sensations, and stay in control of the pain, rather than it controlling you. Just 20 minutes into my first class I had discovered that if I have pain in one part of my body, in this case the twisting arm pain, I could at the very least dull it and, at best, totally block it out by moving my legs. Imagine how you can use this tool in labour; the simplicity of a rhythmic motion like marching or stomping your feet can be used to work through a contraction. It will give you something positive to focus on, a rhythm and movement to help you work through and distract you from the pain.

As you will see from my labour story later in the book and the stories from the other women in this chapter, we each used this technique of movement in our own way to help with the pain during our labours. And for each one of us and countless other women, it worked to change what could have been an unbearable situation into an effective and tolerable one. It is really worth it. Keep yourself moving. Go with it. Match the pain!

My mum came with me to this first class. She was lined up to be my extra support person for my labour and I wanted to know if she believed this method would work as I value her opinions highly – after all, she gave birth four times without any epidurals. I figured she would know how to handle it! Funny thing about my mum coming to class: while I was embarrassed and wanted to hide she was totally into it. She absolutely understood the importance of moving during labour, of freeing up your body to let it do the work.

When Juju asked my mum during class what her labour was like, mum said she was stuck on a bed and told to be quiet as there were other women in the room and they weren't to be frightened. She was not allowed to move. She suffered a bedridden labour four times. She told me how lucky I was to be able to deal with my labour in any way I wanted, in particular being free to move about as and when I felt I needed to. And how lucky we all are to be able to do as we please. This is something we should never forget. Whichever way you give birth, remember how lucky you are to have choices.

I was fortunate that the midwives at The Mater have a lot of Juju's couples and they understand her techniques and encourage them. From the moment I arrived at the hospital, I was encouraged to stay upright and pace back and forth across the delivery room. My first amazing midwife, June (I called her my gym instructor), would come into my labour room and catch me sitting on the end of the bed chatting with my husband and having a cup of tea and a biscuit (I was still in early labour with not much pain). She would make me get off the bed and move around the room, even if it meant I had to carry my cup of tea and biscuit!

I hadn't realised that early labour pain could be quite mild. When my contractions first started at home – they were four minutes apart right from the start – I just relaxed, finished packing my bag and got things ready. My labour pain was so mild at this stage that I didn't need to stop what I was doing during them. This, however, is not the same for everyone as some women have stronger pain from the beginning. One labour can be very different from the next. Even in the car I was happy just chatting with my husband as we drove leisurely to the hospital. Not what I had imagined would be the case!

MARIANTHE *As I entered labour I felt very confident, excited and, above all, at ease. I began using my legs and stomping out the pain at home. While my legs were working my brain was focusing on each and every echo produced by the movement of my feet. When I arrived at the hospital I was 4 centimetres dilated. I continued using my stomping but needed the stress balls as well. At about 7 centimetres I gave my body a rest and changed my technique to my voice as the main means of release, using a focal point on the curtain. The midwife was very supportive and I didn't feel inhibited at all.*

When I arrived at the hospital and was checked by my obstetrician I was 3 centimetres dilated. You may be wondering what centimetres of dilation means. Don't worry, I had no clue either when I first found out I was pregnant. By the time I was in labour, thanks to Juju, I knew how much dilation roughly equalled how much pain and how far advanced the labour was. Unfortunately for many women, including some of my very close friends, they gave birth not knowing what their bodies were doing. One friend of mine arrived at the hospital, was told her labour wasn't progressing fast enough and went in for an emergency caesarean. When I asked her how dilated she was at that point, she said she didn't think to ask.

'Cervical dilation' is a clinical term that measures the progress of your labour. Your body prepares for labour by producing hormones that make the cervix thin. Once labour begins the thinning cervix starts dilating and it is measured in 1-centimetre increments by the medical team; a cervix is fully dilated at 10 centimetres. For most women, these increments move faster between the 5- and 10-centimetre marks than 0 to 5 centimetres. If you have been in labour for eight hours and are only 5 centimetres dilated, don't start thinking it will be another eight hours until you reach 10 centimetres; it may only be three or four hours, or even one or two. The period up until you are 10 centimetres dilated is called the first stage of labour. After this is the pushing and crowning stage, the second stage of labour, and the incredible moment of the birth of your baby.

At the hospital I walked around my labour room and the maternity unit with my mum. Picture this: I was wearing a bright pink nightie with a hospital gown over the top and my rubber flipflops – not my usual social attire! I stayed on my feet until I was about 5 to 6 centimetres dilated, which is about when my legs were starting to get tired and I really wanted to try something different. I had been in labour now for about six hours and Keith, my obstetrician, broke my waters. Once this happens there is usually an immediate increase in pain. I knew to expect this and so I knew I needed to get more actions going. I had to get bigger than the pain.

I recalled a DVD Juju showed in class of a woman in labour sitting on a fit ball and rocking back and forth, using movement and sound to master her pain. She was leaning against the delivery bed to take the pressure off her back. In deep concentration, she rocked backwards and forwards, making long, quite loud rhythmic 'Aahh' sounds. She was frowning but I could see how in control she was. Her partner was counting the seconds of each contraction for her. They were both in rhythm and in sync. In between contractions she stopped and rested her head on her arms. Sometimes at the end of the contraction she would look up and smile. She seemed so calm, which was not what I thought she would be. I was thinking of all those Hollywood films, you know the ones where the woman is screaming in pain the entire way through her labour, completely out of control!

This image of the woman on the DVD using Juju's techniques so successfully was an extremely strong image for me to use while I was in labour. I remembered how the movement was a way for her to keep her labour progressing and to give herself and her husband a rhythm to work with. Most of all it was an image of a woman deep in labour and in control –

an empowering image for me to hold on to. Juju had taught me that movement is vital not only to help you block the pain but also to assist the baby to move down into the pelvis. In this way the baby pushes down on to the cervix, stimulating the labour further. I learned that lesson and used the exact motion the woman in the DVD used for the majority of my labour.

I wanted to rest my legs so sitting on a fit ball worked really well for me. However, because my range of movement decreased in doing so, I needed to match the pain, which was increasing. This is where I brought in vocalisation (see Skill # 2) and I used it the entire time I was on the fit ball and for the rest of the first stage of my labour. I went from 5 to 8 centimetres using these methods. My husband was timing the seconds of each contraction, which helped to keep me focused on something constructive. So I was concentrating on the movement and the sound of my voice and I had my husband keeping me focused on the positive progression of the contraction – I had a beginning, middle and end. In this way, we were working together as a team and I had his voice reassuring me all the way through it.

It's funny. If I think back to how I imagined myself in labour before Juju's classes it was certainly not walking around the room, or rocking on a fit ball, or making loud vocal sounds! I saw myself on the bed calmly dealing with it. I had no idea how I was actually going to achieve that, but I figured I always had the epidural option to fall back on if I didn't cope. Now I know there is no way I could have done it without Juju's preparation. I would have lasted a few hours, maybe, and then become scared by the size of the pain, and then begged for it to stop. What I actually had was a labour where I was in complete control, aware of and ready for my body's monumental changes.

Each time my obstetrician popped into the room he commented on how well I was coping and how in control I was. He watched as my husband and I worked together, as a team. Later he told me he admired our relationship – he was quite moved by the way we worked together through the ups and downs of my labour. It shows how positive an active labour can be for you and for your partner.

By the time I reached 8 to 9 centimetres I had been in labour for about 12 hours. It was feeling extremely powerful and I was exhausted. I needed to lie down but, again, in doing so I needed to match the pain with other skills. I concentrated on touch and sound. Even though I was on the bed I couldn't stop moving as my body felt like it was bursting with energy. I spontaneously went with it. There was no way I could be still. I kept moving my legs back and forth on the sheets while holding on to my husband's shirt, rhythmically crunching it up in the palms of my hands. These sensations, of the sheets under my legs and of the fabric between my fingers, gave me sensory activities to focus on to distract me from the pain and to stay in control.

BROOKE *All morning I had been pacing the floor in my apartment so I found the car ride to the hospital unbelievably restricting. The only way I could endure the journey was to have my husband stop the car at the side of the road just as the contraction was about to start. I then got out of the car and paced along the footpath, comforted by the sight of our car following slowly alongside the kerb. When the contraction ceased I got back into the car until the next one. Then we would repeat the whole process again. It took a little longer to get to the hospital, but at least I mastered the pain.*

For each woman labour pain is different. Contractions are usually isolated to one area, as it was with me, the most common area being the low to mid abdomen, but you may have pain in your back more than your tummy. You may also have pain in your thighs. For all women, though, labour pain grows to be big, really big.

I often think about women whose movement is restricted during labour; those that have to be induced and need constant monitoring for example. Some women do not feel like moving during labour; their legs may feel shaky or tired. This may be you. For every woman there will be moments when you can't move during labour, say when your midwife or obstetrician is checking your cervix for labour progression, or when you have to go to the bathroom. Whatever the situation you will need backup. Just having the various movement techniques Juju teaches on standby whenever you feel like using them is invaluable.

I left this first class feeling energised and inspired. Gosh, before this class I really didn't understand labour pain and I really didn't understand what I was capable of at all. Afterwards I saw my body in a completely new light. I felt empowered by this knowledge and ready to take on my biggest challenge: the birth of my baby. I immediately called my husband when I got home – he was overseas at the time – as I wanted to explain to him what I had learnt. He actually understood what I was talking about, the methodology of mastering pain. He compared it to an athlete working through extreme pain in competition. They have techniques – visualisation, breathing, vocalisation – to get them through it. It made so much sense to both of us. I knew I'd be going back to Juju's classes the next week.

KYLIE *At 6 p.m. I was induced as I had had mild contractions all day but nothing much was happening in terms of progress. The induced contractions came about every two and a half to three minutes. Being attached to the drip was not a problem – the stainless steel stand it was on had wheels so I was not restricted in any way. I began with hip swaying and thigh rubbing with one hand. We walked up and down the length of the room and when this was no longer adequate to manage the pain I moved into the shower and started stomping and using the 'Aahh' sound. The pain was absolutely manageable using these techniques. I felt as though I was releasing the pain through my mouth and down through my feet.*

Think about this idea of using movement to distract from pain and think about where you or your partner may have used it before without realising it. You may have been at the gym, working through an exercise that was painful but you maintained a rhythm and counted the repetitions to work through the pain. Or you may have sprained your ankle and kept moving, shouting 'Ouch' while you flapped your arms about, anything to distract you from the pain. If so, you have already used movement in those parts of your body not in pain to distract your mind from those parts that are. If not, try it next time you experience pain – even mild pain – you might be amazed by the results.

LIZ *Initially, I walked around the maternity section of the hospital with my husband. After an hour or so, we returned to the birthing suite as the pain was increasing, and I wanted to be in my own environment with all my things. I preferred to stay in one position, swaying my hips from side to side and focusing on my body weight as it fell over each foot. After another hour or so my legs started shaking so my midwife and husband put down floor mats and beanbags and I got down on my knees and leaned against the bed.*

SONIA *In early labour I dealt with the contractions by leaning on a bench or chair, swaying my hips from side to side and focusing on my breathing, which was in rhythm with my hip movements. On admission to the hospital I was 4 to 5 centimetres dilated. In my room I found something to lean over, still standing and swaying my hips rhythmically and lifting each leg as I swayed during the contractions. I used some lavender oil on a tissue to help me relax in the new environment and I continued to focus on my breathing and swaying and then the leg lifting. I added a heat pack to my abdomen and my husband massaged my back and my sides for as long as the pain lasted. I also had some music playing, which I used for my swaying rhythm.*

JO *As it was, I was on the bed for the whole labour. My baby was showing some mild signs of distress and I had to be monitored all the time. This meant I couldn't use the bath, the shower, the fit ball or standing, walking or stomping, in fact any of the things I had planned. I knew I had to adapt to the pain by modifying the things I had learned. My main technique was kicking my feet up and down on the bed I was lying on. This felt surprisingly good. I was totally focused on the movement of my legs as well as the slight burning feeling on the skin of my feet that the movement on the sheet created. I also focused on the sound of my heels on the sheets. All of this took my mind off the pain and changed my situation from unbearable to tolerable and workable.*

DIANA *I knew the day we practised legwork for labour contractions that it would be the activity I would use. It just felt right. I didn't like the idea of lying down waiting for the pain to engulf me. As it turned out I could not lie down or even sit down for contractions during both my births. I had to stay mobile. Anything else was absolutely not an option. Barefooted, I stomped up and down the delivery room using the 'Aahh' sound. I was totally focused, totally uninhibited and totally in command of the pain. It worked brilliantly. My husband helped by reminding me I was 'cutting in' too late on some contractions; this reminded me to greet the beginning of the next contraction instantly with leg movements. Sometimes when I looked like I might be losing it he would count me in three seconds before the contraction started: 'Three, two, one … go!' This was even better. I could not begin to imagine what labour would have been like if I could not have used my legs in this way.*

JANET *If anyone had told me years ago that my main technique for coping with first stage labour pain was to submerge my body in water and bang my heels against the foot of the bath, I would not have believed them. My legs worked hard for every contraction over a three-hour period, splashing water everywhere – I must have looked like Tarzan wrestling with an alligator. My* husband was drenched and he had stripped down to his boxer shorts. It may seem a strange thing to do in a top private hospital, but it really did work. By focusing on the kicking my attention was taken away from the pain of each contraction and I felt I had an entirely appropriate activity to express my pain and stress and tension. My midwife was a saint; she just said, 'Go for it,' and I dilated from 2 to 8 centimetres in three hours!

CATHY   *At the beginning of each contraction at home, my husband would repeat the mantras from our classes: 'Pain means action' and 'Keep moving'. This kept me totally focused. The rocking from side to side progressed to stomping with repetitive 'blow' breathing, the sort of breath you use if you're blowing a small ladybird off your arm ... not too hard, not too soft. In the car I stomped my feet and hit stress balls together like cymbals – I must have looked quite peculiar as my husband ordered a quick breakfast at the local drive-through. At the hospital I got down on all fours due to back pain and used my legs to kick against two pillows on the floor. I alternated this with the side-lying position, rubbing one leg against the other while hitting the stress ball on the floor mattress. I found the greatest relief by intensifying the stomping. I was amazed that my lower abdomen was swamped in pain but my legs moved freely, swiftly and lightly. This felt good and I felt very much in control. As I entered transition I got into the bath on all fours, kicking my legs, hitting a stress ball on the edge of the bath and releasing a loud 'Aahh' sound to help with the increasing pain. It was incredible how I could play such an active role in my labour and not just be reduced to a terrified victim wishing it would all just disappear.*

Remember: **Focus on the legs, not the pain.**

A final thought ...

The open and flexible attitude of obstetric professionals is to be admired as women gain more and more freedom in expressing their pain. Be guided by their advice, especially if they observe you are fatiguing yourself and would benefit from a gentler, more restful approach for a while.

Don't use your legs too early in labour. If possible, reserve this active use of the legs until you really need them. You may waste much-needed energy reserves if you stomp around your bedroom during early labour at midnight, and you will probably feel ridiculous as well! Wait until your pain demands you use your more active resources and remember to combine the use of your legs with one or two other birth skills when needed, stopping leg work altogether if appropriate.

In labour your legs can help you to master your pain, just as they did for the women quoted above, but it may not be your preference. The legs, the feet and the hips are only one adaptation choice to help block pain. Use other birth skills if the legs are not right for you, and add others when you need. Perhaps you will benefit more from the birth skills in the next class, 'Breathing and vocalising'.

SKILL # 2

Breathing and vocalising

What is the purpose of teaching you how to use your breath and sound in the first stage of labour?

Simple: pain makes you hold your breath! If you hold your breath in the first stage of labour you make the pain worse, and this book is all about making the pain better.

Breathing and vocalising are natural responses to pain – any pain. With sick pain, sound will take the form of groaning, moaning, screaming, complaining, etc., and the breath is uneven and out of control. With healthy pain you tend to breathe and vocalise rhythmically. In many activities, developing a rhythm is vital to doing a difficult activity. Think about running a marathon or the traditional cultural songs or chants that help a group of people maintain a rhythm so they can do a challenging job – the African Americans in the deep south were adept at this when they laboured in the cotton fields or in a prisoner 'chain gang': the rhythm and sounds helped them through their difficult and painful situation. The chant decreased the spaces of time the workers had to think about the negative aspects of the work they were doing – brilliant! With the placement of value on intellectual supremacy in our society we may well have forgotten about, or even devalued, this simple yet clever tool.

You can do it

In my programme I conduct one class on breath and pain and another one on sound and pain. I do these classes separately because many of my clients book into the programme with the objective of learning 'the breathing', but not necessarily the sound. They are not sure what the breathing is, but they have heard about it and they just know that they want to learn it. Many of their mothers also recommend they learn it because that is what they did when they had their own babies – the Lamaze method of breathing has been part of almost every American sitcom we have seen. They've heard about it as well because rhythmic breathing is incorporated in Pilates programmes, it is in vogue in prenatal yoga classes, and the hypnobirthing trend (a self-hypnosis style) has introduced its own form of breathing suggestions for labour. But going one step further and using sound can also be an incredibly useful tool in blocking labour pain; in fact the title of my vocalisation class is 'Sound Blocks Pain' – and it really does (just read Sarah's section later; she certainly agrees with me)!

JO *I was in the zone, just as you'd described it, and I really wasn't noticing anything around me. This is because I was so focused on the task at hand, that of emptying out my stress and pain through sound. This is all I focused on. As I made my outward 'Aahh' sound I just thought , 'Pain out, Panic out,' over and over again until each 60-second bout of pain was gone.*

Many women are a little shy about my vocalisation class so I like to spend as much time as possible on both the theory and the practice of this auditory skill. Usually, they have inhibitions because sound is often prejudged as unsociable and embarrassing, and something to be avoided for those reasons. We are so prejudiced about any behaviour that is a little out of the ordinary and forget that it might be exactly what we need on the day.

No one seems to have the same inhibitions about breathing quietly, but using only quiet breathing can create another problem; it may be helpful for the mild to moderate pain, but for many women it may not be enough to help with the intense pain, and then you just set yourself up for losing control. It's all very well to learn breath control exercises, but if they don't control the pain, they are useless. Breath control for a yoga stretch or pose, for example, is not the same as breath control for labour pain.

JAYNE *I began by breathing quietly while I listened to Pachelbel, which I found extremely calming. I was 10 days overdue, had an IV drip in my arm, and the contractions were coming every minute. After two hours I was exhausted and must say I was enduring the contractions rather than mastering them. I knew I had to progress to sound if I was going to cope. I gained solace from yelling 'Aahh' rhythmically. I'm sure I could be heard all over Sydney and all the way down to the Opera House. But boy, did it help! And no one cared, least of all me. The midwives were fantastic and so supportive. I focused on the 'Aahh' sound and yelled louder and louder to outdo myself!*

Why do I combine the skills here?

For the purpose of this book, I am combining breath and sound into one chapter as I believe both are universal birthing behaviours that are extremely powerful and as old as time itself. No one invented them, and anyone who says they did when offering birthing advice is kidding themselves. Just consider a newspaper quote by Australian singer Danielle Spencer at the end of her first pregnancy – it made me laugh. A newspaper journalist asked her if she had gone to antenatal classes to 'learn the breathing'. Her response was brilliant: 'I know how to f___ing breathe.' She was spot on! We all do know how to breathe. We have been doing it since birth. We do it when we are awake, when we are asleep, and it adjusts automatically depending on the situation – when running, thinking, painting, laughing, sweeping, yelling, making love, skiing, whispering, blow-drying hair, lugging groceries, dramatising, etc. It adjusts itself, we don't have to do or think anything in particular to regulate it (although we can); it just happens.

So what exactly is the breathing for labour?

Well actually it is quite simple. But I'll get to that in a moment.

Don't hold back

Recently, I took in a couple of old relics to show the women of one of my classes. These were two old books. One my mother, also a physiotherapist, used when she was teaching antenatal classes many years ago. Written in the 1950s when labour and birth took place only on a bed, the behaviour it recommended was totally limiting and the main pain technique taught was the breathing. I read out part of it to my class and invited them to try some of the exercises. Here is the first one:

> *With mouth closed, breathe gently in and out, keeping quite loose and letting the abdominal wall rise up with the indrawn breath and drop down with the outgoing one. This must be practised every day, aiming at taking half a minute or more to draw in the breath and then it can be let go.*

Then it goes on to say, 'This exercise is important because the mother's most important work during labour is accomplished by her controlled breathing.' Remember what I said about maybe controlling the breathing but not controlling the pain?

Breathing in for 30 seconds, or 20 seconds, or even half the suggested time – 15 seconds – when you are in excruciating pain is virtually impossible. Just try it. It's not even easy to do when you are not in pain! I asked the women in my class for some feedback and most of them shook their heads in disbelief while others responded with, 'You can't do it!,' 'It creates stress,' 'Impossible' or 'It makes you hold back'. This last response really tells it the way it is. It makes you hold back! But it was all we had as we lay on those beds all those years ago.

Labour is all about letting go. Letting go of stress, letting go of fear, letting go of pain, letting go of panic, letting go of inhibitions, and letting go of breath and sound. Any activity that makes you hold back is the wrong activity. Why? Because it will make the pain worse, increase your stress level, hold back your oxytocin release, slow down your labour, and inhibit your endorphin mobilisation.

Further on in this vintage book there is another gem of a sentence that goes something like this: 'A contraction has wrongly been called labour pain; it is explained on the ground that ignorance creates fear and the fear creates the pain.' Where do I start?

Let me say this once again: labour pain is real pain. The pain is both a feeling sensation within your body and a thinking analysis in your brain. You feel it and think it at the same time. The pain is created by muscle fatigue. To say that it is only due to fear is an indictment of women's ability to own the process of labour and its pain. Labour pain is not based on a negative emotion such as fear! Sure, fear and panic and terror from a lack of understanding and skills can make the pain worse, but it is not the cause of the pain.

I repeat: Labour pain is real pain. It is a normal accessory to a uterine contraction and it is physical – and don't forget healthy! It's yours and you create it!

The second relic I took to my class was a book published in 1958. Now there were definitely some advances in the neuro-physiological concepts of pain perception in this old and tattered number, but again there were some negative principles that I'm sure have been embedded in the psyche of all pregnant women since that time. In the back of the book is outlined a scoring of six criteria for success with the old-style breathing techniques. The first is: 'Excellent. Complete absence of sensation. Constant comfort of the woman who, throughout her labour, acts as during any everyday activity and adapts herself to her contractions without any effort.' The last score was: 'Failure. Woman restless and screams.'

When I read this out to the class, I asked all of the women who had already had a baby to come to the front, face the class and give their opinion of the failure scoring as well as the excellent scoring. Each one had coped with their first labours in different ways and most of their responses for both scores are, unfortunately, delightfully unprintable! You see, without exception, these women worked through their previous labours successfully with restlessness and noise! They used this restless activity and sound to block their pain, to release their stress, to prevent a distressed state, to stay in control, to exert command over each contraction, to master their situation, to feel empowered. Each had a drug-free labour and not one of them saw themselves as a 'failure' as they used their natural coping tools.

Attitudes have changed

Bear in mind, those two books are about 50 years old and you live in the 21st century.

Times have changed.

You, the women, have changed.

Social sets of rules have changed.

Have you seen the old film footage of the Beatles' first trip to Australia? It created history in terms of mass hysteria for pop stars; although my mother told me it was pretty wild when a chap called Johnnie Ray came to Sydney in the 1950s! (Ask your grandparents about this one.) Do you realise that those very same women, who were screaming, yelling, crying in joy and ecstasy, emptying themselves of stress, excitement, love, pain, trying to break down barricades to reach the Fab Four, were the very same women who, just a few years later, had their babies while lying on their backs, suffering in silence? I do: I was one of them.

Crazy!

You can be different, put your breath to work and make it work harder than the pain. Put your sound to work, focus on it and make it work for you to block your pain.

BRIGID *I 'Aahhed' and 'Aahhed' much louder than I ever thought I was capable of. I focused on the sound of my voice and paced around the coffee table. The pain felt so minimal that I kept thinking, 'It must get worse than this.' When I got to the hospital I was fully dilated. I felt in such command and control. I was confident and felt no fear. I now tell all my friends, 'Sound blocks pain and you can do it'!*

Those limited breathing exercises and passive relaxation techniques are out of date. They were designed to try to help women who laboured only on their backs and only on a bed. Let's face it, if that's all you were permitted to do, you had to be creative with the only thing you had going for you: breath and the mental ability to try to relax. But those breathing techniques were too hard and had a low success rate; they were more of a performance than a tool.

Whatever you do to prepare for the birth, make sure you equip your-selves with a range of activities. If you choose the gentler approach (yoga breathing, hypnobirthing, calm birthing, gentle birthing) and it does not work effectively for you on the day, make sure you have learned more active skills as a backup to use in their place. Different things work for different people; the problem is that no one knows until the day what will work. Try not to approach the education for your labour with an either/or mentality. Learn everything. Practise everything.

I still teach the breathing and relaxation techniques I taught over 30 years ago but they are now only one part of the preparation section in my course. I find it really powerful to begin my breathing class with excerpts from those two precious old relics, which I have to keep in tissue paper and a plastic bag. They help every member of the class gain insight into the breathing as an historical phenomenon, and also understand how the social sets of rules of yesteryear in delivery suites are no longer appropriate or even expected today. The breathing is different now. You can combine it with limitless creative activity. It is more spontaneous rather than tightly controlled. It is much, much better.

And easier!

MICHAELA   *It was 13 paces from one wall of the delivery suite to the other. My husband and I paced up and down together, both blowing towards a power point on one end and the logo on my sports bag at the other. He helped me focus and concentrate on the task at hand. As the pain built up, I kept 'blow-breathing' while my husband started counting one to 13 with each step, back and forth across that room for six hours! It is exactly what got us through.*

A little physiology ...

The breathing in labour is a little like the breathing for an exercise workout, but not exactly. The breath *in* provides oxygen for you and the baby and the muscle needed for the birth activity, and the breath *out* takes away the carbon dioxide, the stress and the tension created by the contraction. All you need to think about, basically, is using your *outward* breath to release all of this. Think: 'Release'; and feel: 'Release', as you do this.

The inward breath mostly looks after itself, and some women find it useful to visualise dilation as this happens. Every time a painful established contraction comes just open your mouth and empty your body of breath, sound and pain, and therefore stress. You may use a slower, more controlled breath (much slower and more controlled than the breath you are using as you read this text), consciously making it as slow as possible if you choose, but only if this works for you. It is your personal preference. Otherwise, let it go. If you do use a very slow, controlled breath you will have to focus on the breath to the exclusion of everything else. You will have to see it in your mind, listen to it, concentrate on it as it comes in through your nostrils and out through your lips, put every ounce of effort into keeping it calm, thinking calm thoughts, unlocking it when the pain wants to immobilise it, and making sure you avoid hyperventilation at the same time. But then it may not work even if you have practised it throughout pregnancy.

Breath, and sound, during labour should reduce pain and *release* stress, not make it worse. When you read the excerpts from the women's labour reports later you will find that in most cases this is what happens. Generally, I find that only about 10 per cent of the women in my classes remain with a quieter form of breathing release throughout all of the first stage of labour; the other 90 per cent, in order to stay in control, need to progress at some point from quiet breathing to audible vocalisation to block the pain – usually the 'Aahh' sound but some sing, talk, hum, moan, groan, etc.

JENNI *Before my husband arrived at the delivery suite I was feeling very inhibited about mastering the pain. I was embarrassed and shy and was internalising my pain response – just the opposite of what I had been taught to do. When he arrived, everything changed, thank goodness. With his encouragement I started to vocalise and release the pain, an enormous relief and so effective. Instead of bottling it all up, I now let it all go. We spent four hours together in the shower, with my husband talking me through and saying the sounds with me. I found making the noise a most amazing release. I couldn't not make the noise. At one stage, I was listening to all the sounds I was making with fascination, exploring different tones and pitches. I look back now and realise that as I listened to my own sound, I did not focus on the pain. In fact, as long as I did this, I could not feel the pain.*

Breath, which includes variations of inhalation, exhalation and blowing and panting, and sound are used as vehicles to empty out the stress and tension from your body during contractions. The breath can be focused on during the contractions (so that you don't concentrate on the pain) and can also calm you and help you centre yourself in between the contractions. Remember, for most women there is no pain in between the contractions. At this time you do nothing. Breathe normally. Breathe calmly.

Vocalisation can be used to match the pain, mobilise your endorphins and create a really loud non-painful rhythmic focus to help you distract from the intense pain. You are neurophysiologically equipped to do this. 'Match the pain' means overriding the uterine pain stimuli with the 'Aahh' sound stimuli in order to change your brain's perception of the original uterine pain. In other words, you make your 'Aahh' so loud that you don't notice the pain – think trumpets and all the other brass instruments in an orchestra. And don't forget to focus on the sound of your own sound.

Remember, breathing and vocalising:

- deplete adrenalin so they are great when you're freezing in fear
- produce endorphins so they are excellent for pain
- produce a wonderful non-painful rhythmic focus to concentrate on
- provide a rhythmic release that helps block panic
- are a wise and clever choice for pain management.

Putting it all into practice

Now let's get really specific. I am going to walk you through the first stage of labour. It will provide some structure for you but this is not a recipe, only a guide. Practise these steps throughout your pregnancy and alter them as you need. There are many, many variations to them.

- In early labour, whether it's during the day or in the middle of the night, you will be reasonably passive, just doing what you would normally be doing, and maybe not even taking too much notice of your contractions if they are only at the level of mild period pain. The sort of breathing you will be doing is the sort of breathing you are doing right now, as you read this.

- As your labour builds up a little, even though you are still at home, you may change your breathing slightly, to make it a little slower so that it becomes a tool you can concentrate on. You will probably sit down, or lean over a bench or an armchair or a table for the duration of the contraction, or even pace slowly up and down the hallway. You will continue with this soft, passive form of breathing. You will concentrate on this breathing (focus on the breath in, focus on the breath out) and you will use it to relax, to release, to let go, particularly during the breath out. Of course, step it up if you need to.

- If you are showering at home, use the same breathing for the contraction as well as maintaining a swaying action as the warm water sprays over your abdomen. Let your body go floppy and see what sort of breathing you do naturally. Try this for a while. Use the 'Aahh' sound if you need.

- As your labour builds up a little more, experiment with different rates and rhythms of breathing to see which suits your pain at the time. Just focus on the in and out, the in and out, the in and out ... Try to maintain that floppy rag doll feeling if possible, at least on the outward breath. Releasing stress is vital.

- In the car on your way to the hospital, try to keep your breath as soft and as slow and as relaxed as possible while you listen to your partner talk or count. You may prefer to listen to some relaxing music. You may include a tissue with essential oils. You may have a heat pack on your abdomen and, of course, use sound as and when you need it.

- In the car park, lobby and lift, just do your best to keep breathing rhythmically. Try to stay calm. This can be a very stressful time as you are moving from the home territory of your car to the hospital. Be aware that your breathing by this time could be more of a 'blow' (like blowing dust away) rather than a breath. This is good. It will probably be more active than passive. Many women have changed to sound by this time, but see how you go.

- When you arrive you will be welcomed by your midwife and have your admission checks. This may include a 20-minute period of monitoring when you will be required to be on a bed – you won't be here long. Don't just lie there fretting. Keep breathing, add sound if you need it. Add stress balls or visualisation or counting. Try to relax through this 20-minute check. Your 60-second contractions (and you may have none during this check-up) will pass quickly if you are busy. Then get up and move about, use your legs.

- Your labour will start escalating and you will no doubt be introducing other skills at this time, so breathing or vocalising (try 'Aahh' or 'Oww') will be only one of several things you do to block the pain. Remember to match the pain. If you need to get louder, do it. Crank it right up! Relax your throat as you do this.

- Do you need a change of scenery, perhaps? Take yourself into the shower. Take a fit ball if it fits in the cubicle. Breathe and bounce, and vocalise and visualise and focus. By now, breathing may be a minor activity and other birth skill tools could be the ones you are focusing on. But keep the breathing going, rhythmically and at the right pace for you. If you are vocalising, keep it rhythmic also, and remember to keep the breath in short, but push the sound out as long or as short as you need. You won't know the pace or volume until the moment, and the length of your breath and sound will vary throughout your labour. If you are in a bath or a spa, blow at a candle propped on the bath edge; if you are not able to light it, no problem, just stay focused on blowing at the wick.

- Eventually you will be using your breath or sound to keep other parts of yourself rhythmic. Everything will be active: breathing, vocalising, legs, hips, hands, eyes, nose, thoughts, keywords, mantras, whatever choices you make to help you stay in command of the pain. Adrenalin gives you the energy to do all of this. You may not be using all these parts of yourself: just know it's all right if you want to. Again, you won't know what you will need until the day.

- When you reach the second stage of labour the breathing changes again, but I'll teach you all about that in Skills # 6 and # 7.

Do it your way

However you use the skills of breath and sound think of emptying your-self of the stress, pain, panic, fear, anxiety and anything else that contributes to a frozen, frightened state. That's what these skills are for. Stay focused on this. A good analogy is to think of yourself as being a vacuum cleaner in reverse – just turn on the switch and out it goes! Blow all that painful dust away! Come on, blow!

You do not have to make the breath do anything you don't want it to do. You don't have to let it in or out for any given number of seconds. Don't even try. If you do anything with your breath that causes more pain or more stress then change the way you are breathing. Remember at the beginning of this chapter when I told you how the breath adjusts to any given situation? Try to work as much as possible with the natural flow of your breathing. During pregnancy you can practise your breathing and vocalising as part of your exercise programmes, in a deep state of relaxation, while working, and with the breathing skills exercises from this book. In labour it will be slow, moderate, fast, whatever is right at the time.

There is one thing that you may not be prepared for when you are in labour and I want to say it again so you understand the concept: *Pain makes you hold your breath and holding your breath makes your pain worse.*

This is why the breathing is useful.

This is why you need to use it to help you relax and let go.

You need to stay focused on keeping the breath flowing in and out, in and out, in and out, in and out … always putting the focus on the *outward* breath. Use the breath to release the stress.

NICOLE *Immediately after an acupuncture session my contractions began at six minutes apart. I lay there on my side and just breathed through my contractions using the hummingbird breathing I had learned at yoga classes. We spent the next three hours at home with me kneeling on a pillow with my arms draped over the fit ball. I was breathing deeply and slowly, feeling I was releasing all my tension and fear each time I exhaled. By the time I arrived at the hospital, I had combined my loud exhalation with the repetitive 'Aahh' sound. This became louder and louder in order to match the pain. Matching the pain was very much a part of my focus. In order to do this I had to close my eyes throughout each contraction. I was vaguely aware of the lemon oil in the burner and sipped raspberry leaf tea and water in between the contractions.*

Sounds easy, doesn't it?

If labour pain stayed only at the level of period pain, it would be easy. But it builds and builds and builds, and as it builds it gets harder and harder to freely breathe in and out, in and out, in and out. That's the beauty of adding other birth skills and engaging your partner in it.

Remember the wonderful and joyful ways everyone celebrated as their team won a match in the World Cup football competition (and the negative expression of stress when games were lost)? In Federation Square in Melbourne alone, trumpets were played, whistles were blown, car horns were tooted, and supporters were yelling, singing and cheering, among other noisy activities. I also had to laugh with enjoyment when the television showed incredible images of fans in Italy turning their famous fountains into splashing playpens as they jumped while yelling, blowing horns, singing and rejoicing! What were all these people doing? Freely expressing their stress – positive or negative.

Stress is designed to be externalised, not kept inside. Keep that in mind for labour, and use your breath and sound wisely to achieve this.

Breathing skills

Let's do it! These exercises are not prescribed techniques for labour, but rather short, 60-second practice sessions to help you become familiar with your breath, and to help you understand how vision, sound, feeling, thought and action interrelate with breath during contractions. It will be interesting to see where your natural focus falls. To add some stress hold a piece of ice as you practise and try to distract yourself from the cold. This increases your tolerance of enduring something that gets beyond just aggravating.

WATCHING YOUR BREATH

Observe the natural flow of your breath. First the inward breath and then the outward breath. Just 'look' at it. Imagine you are breathing through an early labour contraction. Work with the flow of this imaginary contraction with this focused watching of your breath. Just relax and look at the flow of your breath as it flows naturally. **Concentrate only on the breath, not the pain**.

LISTENING TO YOUR SOUND

Repeat the same activity, this time focusing on the sound of your breath. Allow the breath to flow comfortably in and out of your nose and mouth or just your mouth. Breathe through your contraction listening to your breath. Just relax and listen to your breath as it flows naturally. **Concentrate only on the breath, not the pain**.

ADD A 'YES'

Follow your normal breathing rate and say to yourself 'Yes' each time you breathe out. In labour this can mean anything you want it to. It can mean 'Yes, cervix open', it can mean 'Yes, I can do this', it can mean 'Yes, I need to stay open' or 'Yes, I can trust this contraction' or 'Yes,

I know exactly what is going on inside my body' or 'Yes, this contraction will soon be over'. Start thinking a 'Yes' ... then whisper the 'Yes' ... then say a 'Yes'. **Concentrate only on the breath, not the pain**.

'OPEN' UP

Focus on the *inward* breath and think 'Open'. Feel the inward breath and feel 'Open'. Hear the inward breath and say to yourself 'Open'. Then exhale normally, and relax. Then do this on the outward breath. Which one do you prefer? Keep this in mind for labour. Is your 'Open' mantra easier with the breath 'in' or the breath 'out'? **Concentrate only on the breath, not the pain**.

WORKING THE WORDS

Try a combination of word imagery with the breath in and relaxation with the breath out. With each breath in think 'Open', with each breath out think 'Release'.

Note: In labour, this might be too complex, but try it anyway.

Progress to just focusing on the word 'Release' with the breath out, and forget about the breath in, just let it happen naturally. **Concentrate only on the breath, not the pain**.

BLOW IT ALL AWAY

Observe your breath as you blow gently through pursed lips. Feel how your lips are placed. Feel the air as it moves past your lips. Relax your lips as you breathe in again. As you blow out again, hear the sound of the escaping breath. Focus on this.

Note: Blowing through pursed lips will become more important than simple breathing through relaxed lips for many of you.

Add another step: Close your eyes and imagine you are blowing a little paper boat across a pond. Breathe in and blow that boat a little further. Now imagine you are blowing a feather. Keep blowing, and keep imagining.

Add another step: Now blow through an imaginary circle about 25 centimetres away from you. Aim to blow the circle wider (visualise your cervix opening and ask your partner to verbalise 'Cervix open'). Or aim to blow your tension through the circle. Empty the stress out of your body and blow it into the circle. Think 'Clean it out', or 'Clear it out', or 'Empty it out', or 'Let it go'. **Concentrate only on the breath, not the pain**.

TOO SOON TO PUSH

There may come a point when you have the urge to push and it is too early to do this. Practise this breathing to pull back from a premature pushing urge. Get down on all fours or lie on your side. Pant, focusing *outwards*, as fast as you need to. The objective is to stop yourself pushing downwards. Focus on panting out to prevent yourself from pushing down – it's hard to do both together. **Concentrate only on the breath, not the pain**.

Guidelines for breathing

- Focus mainly on the outward breath.
- Don't over-control it and don't under-control it.
- Concentrate on associated imagery, such as blowing out a candle at all paces and rhythms.
- Adapt your breathing routines to suit your pain, such as the breaths you already know, like when swimming, doing yoga or Pilates, walking, meditating, etc.
- The objective is to breathe to control the pain – the breath is pain free, the contraction hurts, don't forget this.
- You will and should forget about your breath totally if you are deeply focused on something else. It will probably happen naturally.
- At all times try to keep it rhythmic, no matter what pace you are breathing.

Caution: hyperventilation

This occurs when there is an imbalance of oxygen and carbon dioxide. You can experience physical signs of dizziness or numbness in the fingers and toes and blueness in the lips. If you feel this, breathe into your own cupped hands or a small paper bag and calm your breath as much as possible. Try to change your skill to vocalisation, as it is almost impossible to hyperventilate using sound.

Vocalising skills

The 'Aahh' sound is no big deal. It is nothing to be inhibited about. It is a little like the 'Aahh' sound you make when you go to the doctor with a sore throat. We've all done it. A doctor says, 'Open wide,' and we do. He then says, 'Now say "Aahh" for me,' and we do as he looks into our throats. In labour, you will be using the same sound over and over again (or similar variations on this theme), and louder and louder, until the contraction has gone. Then you rest, your baby rests, and your partner rests as well. Let's try it.

Vocalisation guidelines for the woman

- Relax your throat.
- Be as loud as you need.
- Vocalise only during the contraction, not in between.
- Vocalise only on the outward breath, not on the short breath in.
- Return to quiet, slow breathing for a while if you get tired.
- Ask your partner to join in.
- Listen to him and focus on his voice.
- Combine sound with other skills, for example visualisation, keywords.

Vocalisation for the partner

- Encourage her to use it to the max – it's part of our fight/flight reflex.
- Remind her it is natural, it's universal – she is not to be embarrassed.
- If she is losing control say, 'Louder!' – this is instantly empowering.
- Vocalise with her.
- Explore different sounds with her.
- For her to turn her pain down, you must encourage her to turn herself up.

THE 'AAHH' SOUND

Think of a newborn baby, and say 'Aahh,' as in, 'Isn't she cute.' This is a soft, gentle, natural sound. Observe your natural 'Aahh' sound. Notice its releasing, letting-go effect. **Focus on the sound of your sounds, not the pain**.

VARY THE RHYTHM

Make your 'Aahh' sound long and relaxed, then short and sharp. **Focus on the sound of your sounds, not the pain**.

SEE A MESSAGE

Practise your sounds with powerful images in your mind, such as 'baby down' or 'climbing stairs'. Do this while your partner counts 'One, two' to give you a rhythm. **Focus on the sound of your sounds, not the pain**.

THINK A MESSAGE

Practise your 'Aahh' sound with mental messages, such as 'Pain out', or 'Stress out', as you say it.
Add another step: Increase the volume of your 'Aahh' and think 'power' – you can harness this power.

Add another step: Repeat your 'Aahh' sound again and think to yourself, 'Aahh blocks pain.'

Note: You can harness the power of the meaning of these words with your 'Aahh' during labour.

Experiment with variations of the 'Aahh' sound. **Focus on the sound of your sounds, not the pain**.

MAKE IT A TEAM EFFORT

Practise making the 'Aahh' sound with your partner and draw on the power of the two of you together. **Focus on the sounds of your sounds, not the pain**.

THROW AWAY THOSE INHIBITIONS

Close your eyes and see yourself as a healthy woman with a healthy sound entirely appropriate to blocking labour pain. Say 'Aahh' like you mean it and own it and what others think about it doesn't matter. **Focus on the sound of your sounds, not the pain**.

SEND IT OUT

Now think of distance – the next room in your house, outside your house, down the street, three blocks away – and make your sound travel that far. In labour, you might need to be thinking three suburbs away! **Focus on the sound of your sounds, not the pain**.

SOUND FOR TRANSITION

When you practise panting in preparation for that very strong pushing urge during transition make it a noisy pant to make it more effective – you are nearly there! **Focus on the sound of your sounds, not the pain**.

A lesson from *The Little Prince*

Sometimes, in my classes, I refer to Antoine de Saint-Exupéry's story and the Little Prince's dedication to 'cleaning out his volcanoes'. In the story the Little Prince tells the reader how he 'cleans out his active volcanoes as well as his inactive volcanoes'. He says if volcanoes are well cleaned out, they 'burn slowly and steadily, without any eruptions'.

I want you to think about this concept for a moment. Under the visible part of a natural volcano we know that there is a combination of heat and energy, magma and lava, and the movement of the tectonic plates. Sometimes to release the pressure the volcano only smokes, at other times when the pressure is greater it bursts fire, sometimes it needs to belch out lava and sometimes, when there is enormous activity beneath the earth's crust, it erupts with everything it has.

Now think for a moment about the activity beneath your abdominal surface in labour. There is heat and energy, movement and stress, pressure and pain. Your project is to release it. Just like a little volcano. Just like the Little Prince with his volcanoes, if you clean out your stress slowly and steadily throughout labour – breathing and blowing and 'Aahhing' it away – hopefully you will never get to 'erupt' (lose control).

If the inside activity is small, you will need to empty gently only, if at all. As it builds, you will have to work at emptying more. And more often. As it increases in intensity even more you will have to focus on many ways of emptying including a variety of skills. As the Little Prince says, 'keep cleaning out as you go' and you will never get to erupt, or as we so often say 'lose control'. 'Cleaning out your contractions' – an unusual way of thinking about pain mastery, but a brilliant way to keep you focused on the task at hand!

JENNIFER *I combined breathing with messages in my head of 'cleaning' and 'clearing'. I just kept thinking of clearing out the pain. It worked brilliantly. It was very simple but very focused. Very disciplined. Just like the Little Prince!*

And now Sarah has a wonderful story to tell you about how she and her husband used sound to block the pain of contractions. I love reading her story as I love to bring together the image of the Sarah I know on a day-to-day basis, and the Sarah who worked so well with her husband in labour – both the same woman, but two very different images.

Sarah's story

After learning how to use movement as a tool to distract from pain I began to realise how important it was to know it, and how wonderful it would be to learn more skills to use during my labour. My next class on the use of the breath and sound began with movement again, all of us marching in our rows across the room. Movement wasn't embarrassing to me anymore as I was now used to it and I knew it worked. But then Juju asked us to add in long, and loud, 'Aahh' sounds. I managed a squeak. Looked around. But, again, no one cared what anyone else was doing.

'Okay, a bit louder,' Juju said. A bit louder? Never in a million years could I have imagined myself standing in a room surrounded by lots of pregnant women making 'Aahh' sounds while marching on the spot! Funny, I also remember thinking there was no way I could see myself marching and making loud 'Aahh' sounds in labour. But I did.

As you can probably tell I am a bit self-conscious and there was no way I was going to bring attention to myself in any public place in any embarrassing way! What if someone heard me? What if my doctor saw me? Wouldn't the midwives laugh? What if people were walking down the hall outside? As my obstetrician, Keith, had highly recommended Juju to me, I knew he was familiar with her techniques so he wouldn't think them silly during my labour. But I knew when the time came I wouldn't feel comfortable enough to do it in front of him. So I had a plan.

I figured if I used the techniques in my labour and he entered the room I would tone them down. The problem with this plan was, once my labour pain got bigger so did my vocalisation and movement. I was in the middle of one contraction and in deep concentration when Keith came in to check on me, so I immediately halved the level of sound and movement I was using to distract from my pain. Whoa!

Instantly I noticed the pain and it began to overwhelm me. I tried to smile at Keith and look confident but I became engulfed in the pain and began to lose control. I had to get back to where I was. I had to get bigger. I had to get back in control. As soon as I found my rhythm and level of sound again with my husband's help, I was back on track and the labour continued on smoothly.

Juju had told us the stress of being out of control, followed by the fear, panic and anger, increases your adrenalin level, which slows down your production of the hormone oxytocin, and consequently slows down labour. The courage and confidence to keep moving and working with the pain increases the flow of oxytocin and moves the labour along. This makes so much sense to me now. I can just see what would have happened if I had laid on my back in bed like my mother had all those years ago. It would have been unbearable and I would have lost control immediately.

Take a bit of time now to think about your labour. Would you rather be lying on a bed, writhing in pain, out of control and hating every second of it, just opting for the epidural right away, or would you rather give it a go by taking action, being positive and staying active throughout your contractions? Juju always said to us that it is not about how long you do the skills during labour, or whether you have a 'natural' birth, or whether you opt for medical help, it is about your experience, your adventure, your labour. But I can say from my experience that even if you try the skills for a short while during labour you will give yourself a chance to be a part of the miracle of birth. I hope this inspires you to give it a go.

There are usually women in Juju's classes who have come back for their second or third labours, which seemed funny to me during my first pregnancy. If they had learned the methods already why were they back for a second or third time? Now, as the due date for my second child approaches, I totally understand it. I have had moments of doubt and coming back for me is like training – you re-familiarise yourself with how to use your body, and through Juju's techniques you re-familiarise yourself with how to manage the pain. There is also the likelihood that my second labour will be very different from my first, which only confirms how important it is to go into labour with as many skills as possible to call upon when and if necessary. Then I can be prepared, totally prepared, for any situation.

I also found that as I now knew what to expect this made labour a bit more daunting but I came back to Juju's classes and felt inspired and positive about the adventure that was to come. My negative feelings went and I began to feel excited. Nervous, yes, but not negative or fearful. It was a wonderful feeling to be excited and to look forward to my labour rather than feel fear and anxiety – defeated before I'd even begun.

For my first labour, in order for us to better understand Juju's techniques, she showed us a DVD of women in labour. I wish you could have seen those women as the images they instil in your mind are wonderful to take into labour. It can be difficult to fully understand when learning in a classroom or reading from a book how the skills work. By watching a woman in labour you can immediately see how effective the skills are and see how they work. This DVD was of a woman in labour in a shower. She was bellowing out long 'Aahh' sounds while her husband was repeating, 'Let it out,' 'Let the pain out,' 'It's healthy pain.' I could see the water pounding on her back, soothing her, but she was a woman in action. She really influenced me as she was in such control.

This immediately removed some of the fear I had of labour pain. Watching this woman staying in control and working through her contractions by using movement and vocalisation completely opened my eyes to different ways to work through labour pain. It helped me see what I could do in my labour. I knew then that my labour was going to be very different from my mum's and all those women who were told to lie on the bed and breathe. I had a new set of images and choices to take with me into that room. I could see what was possible and that I had options.

Some of the other women in Juju's classes, like me, had repeatedly said they never thought they would use vocalisation during labour as they were quiet people, not into attracting attention towards themselves. But in the end they all used it, just as I did. I used the fit ball to rock back and forth for movement and, boy, did I use the vocalisation. As the pain became stronger I kept a rhythm on the ball while my husband counted through the contraction. I felt very much in control.

ANNA *At midnight I was in fairly strong labour and managed by using a heat pack and walking around the living room. Despite holding off for as long as I could, by 1.30 a.m. I needed the 'Aahhs'. My husband encouraged me to focus on my noise and we continued this during the car journey to the hospital. When we arrived an hour later we continued the same sound, but louder. I didn't want the bath, the shower, massage oils or counting – I just needed the freedom to do my 'Aahhs' and have my husband remind me to focus on my noise. This got me all the way through first stage.*

I had also studied yoga throughout the final stages of my first pregnancy with a wonderful midwife/yoga teacher, Maureen. She taught me the importance of relaxing and breathing in between contractions, to rest my body in preparation for the next contraction. I certainly used her techniques; I even used them in the car on the way to the hospital. I wanted to conserve my energy so when I could be still, I would be. This helped me stay in control, clear my mind, and prepare for the next contraction.

Early in my labour, when the pain was quite mild, I didn't need to use sound so much. I was blowing out the pain with just my breath. It was a bit like when you lift a heavy weight at the gym: as any good trainer will tell you, you need to breathe out on the lift. The breath out distracts you from the pain as you lift the weight. It is the same with running or any other sort of aerobic exercise: you keep breathing, rhythmically. I found it was the same with labour. At first my breath was soft but as the contractions increased in intensity, when I was about 4 or 5 centimetres, I increased the strength of the breath – forcefully blowing out the pain. Eventually this wasn't enough and I began to notice the pain. I knew I needed to introduce a new technique, otherwise all I was focusing on was the increasing level of pain.

Juju's vocalisation was, for me, an extension of the breath. At first it was a quiet 'Aahh' sound but it gradually increased and increased in volume to form loud 'Aahh' sounds. It was important that the sounds were rhythmic as this kept me in control. By making long 'Aahh' sounds through each contraction, I was breathing out in forceful long breaths along with it. This forced breathing and the sound of my voice helped me stay calm and in control.

As soon as I brought in the vocalisation and focused my mind completely on the sound the pain disappeared into the background. When I noticed the pain again, I would get louder. The repeated, rhythmic, loud 'Aahh' sound kept me focused on something other than the pain: it forced the pent-up energy out of my body, kept me in control and helped to block the pain. The sound was blocking the pain! As well, I was successfully working off my adrenalin, cranking up the production of endorphins and thereby decreasing my perception of pain (I'm sure they could hear it miles and miles away!) and the midwives were encouraging me to do it. They told me they could tell by my sound how far along in my labour I was. Once I was using louder sound the midwives could see how concentrated I was on each contraction and how focused I needed to be in order to stay in control. They knew the labour was progressing as it should.

As I increased the level of sound I got more and more self-conscious. I was embarrassed. Thank God for my husband. He was shouting, 'Come on, I've heard you louder than that! You can be louder!' His encouragement made me feel it was okay. In my moments of inhibition I knew I would have to give up if I didn't keep using Juju's techniques, so I had to make a decision: give up and get an epidural, or keep going.

As exhausting as the labour was I knew I was experiencing something incredible. This was it. This was my labour. This was the moment I had been building up to my entire life. And I wanted to give it a go. To really give it a go. I wanted to experience the whole thing. It was so exciting. The pain, the ups and downs of the contractions, the midwives coaching me, my doctor encouraging me and my husband supporting me. Each passing hour was another triumph of getting that little bit closer to the birth of my baby. No, I didn't want to numb it down. I wanted to keep going. My husband and I were a team and were working together so well. I had to give myself permission to get over the inhibitions and to really embrace what I was experiencing.

SOPHIE *With a posterior presentation, I was on all fours, had excruciating backache, and my cave woman sound was out in force. She was in her element when I was stuck in transition for two hours. I never thought it possible. The adrenalin really does kick in, doesn't it? (Thank goodness!)*

I brought the vocalisation back in with movement. I refocused on what I was doing and ignored what I thought everyone else was thinking. I never believed I would make the level of noise I made but it was the most natural thing. The use of vocalisation during my contractions took my mind off the pain and brought my focus to the sound of my voice. I could hear the intonations. Sometimes I would go up at the end, 'Aahh-uuhhhhhhhh,' or sometimes the other way around: 'Uuhh-aahhhhhhhh.' Not only was I blocking the pain, I also knew I was producing endorphins to help me through it.

Midwives were walking in and out of my room. My obstetrician, Keith, came in repeatedly to check on me. Did I care who was in the room? Not one bit! The birth skills were helping my pain and I was totally focused. I wouldn't even have cared if George Clooney had walked into the room! Okay, I might have stopped to have a gawk, but this was really how great it was at distracting me! Vocalisation was the only way I could get through my labour in control, with courage, and with confidence. It was everything!

MARIANNE *By the time we got to the hospital I had lost my normal friendliness and my inhibitions had long gone. Candle-blowing breathing was an absolute joke at this point, due to the level of pain, so my husband led me in a slow, rhythmical 'Aahh'. As we did this together he told me to stay in command, to focus on the noise and to stay centred.*

With every contraction this would bring me back to control the noise, rather than falling victim to the hysterical edge that was coming through.

I know most of you reading this are saying, 'There is no way I will use vocalisation in my labour.' Well, I was just like you. And if you read the labour stories in this book most, if not all, of the women who used vocalisation never imagined they would have either. In that moment of labour and childbirth all social parameters do disappear. What seems weird and embarrassing while you are reading this book has no relevance to the time when you will be in labour. No one will mind how you work through your labour pain. In fact, I was encouraged to be active and vocal. What you experience in labour is something so miraculous everything is out of the ordinary. You will see!

DIMITY *At 8 a.m., when my contractions were 20 minutes apart, I rang the hospital and the midwife said to come in when they were five minutes apart. So we relaxed and I simply leaned over the ottoman and did some slow breathing while my husband counted softly every time a contraction came. I imagined I was blowing a tissue; later blowing enough to send a little plastic boat across a lake. The important part was the outward breath, so my husband started counting only on the outward breath, starting at one and going up to eight, slowly progressing from one to four as my breath got shorter and faster in order to handle the pain. We did not go to the hospital for 16 hours. On admission I was told I was only 3 centimetres dilated and had experienced a long pre-labour. I was glad I had used only breathing, imagery and counting as well as a hot pack doused with lavender oil, as I still had a long way to go. I would have been exhausted otherwise. As it turned out our baby was born just six hours later, but I guess one never knows just how long it will be.*

SARA *On arrival at the maternity ward at 1 a.m., the initial examination revealed that I was 3 centimetres dilated. We rang mum, who is 73 years old, and she arrived at 2 a.m. and stayed for the entire labour. She was as supportive to my husband as she was to me. Because I had felt nauseous, we had located a stainless steel bowl in case I vomited, but later it became a good tool for handling pain. Over the next few hours, as the regular contractions continued, I stood, leaning on my elbows over the foot of the bed, stamping and 'Aahhing' away the pain. As I needed to intensify my activity to match the pain, I increased the amplitude of my 'Aahhs' towards the bowl – Juju always told us to turn the dial up! I focused on the sound reverberation within the bowl. This brought added distraction, and emphasised the power of the 'Aahh' sound. It was all I needed.*

KIM *By 7 centimetres, I decided it was time for the shower. The contractions were now very intense and the water provided great relief. I leaned forward, supporting myself on one of the shower bars, rocked, and held the shower nozzle low over my abdomen and back alternatively. My poor husband must have felt like a third leg at this point as I just didn't want anyone else in charge of that nozzle but me! We have laughed about this many times since. I then starting using my voice, which was the greatest relief from the pain. The louder I groaned, the less it hurt. I stood in the shower for about an hour and made the most primal noises I'd ever heard. I'm sure I could not make those noises again, even if I wanted to. They are strong powerful noises that come from deep within. I did not realise I had carried them with me all of my life just waiting for this day. They provide the most unbelievable relief from the pain. After another hour or so in the shower, I got the urge to push.*

LOUISE *Labour was progressing slowly. I was 3 centimetres dilated on admission and four hours later I was only 4 centimetres. I was really disappointed and wondered how on earth I was going to cope. I was exhausted and I found the pain unbearable. The midwife suggested I walk around the maternity ward. Reluctantly I paced the corridors for the next hour. Then, I decided to try the shower and I was in it for about an hour. By this time I was matching the pain and I didn't care who heard me. I was shouting at the top of my voice, 'Aahh,' 'Aahh,' 'Aahh.' My husband was saying it with me and holding the shower hose over my back exactly where I told him to: 'Aahh, higher. Aahh, lower …' I was supporting myself on the wall of the shower with one hand and hitting it as fast as I could with the sponge with the other. I had my eyes shut during the contractions but in the end I had to stare at my sponge hitting the wall. I had my next examination and I was 9 centimetres! An hour later I gave birth.*

SALLY *Labour began at 3.30 a.m. on my due date. I managed the early pain by breathing in and out in a calm, even rhythm. I swayed my hips in time with the rhythm. I walked the garden paths, I rested, I walked again, I snacked, I showered. As the contractions continued with surprising regularity, I realised their message, 'Baby's coming, baby's coming.' This was a comforting mantra, and really exciting. Twenty-four hours later, and three changes of hospital midwives, the contractions finally started to intensify (why didn't I read about pre-labour?) Regulated breathing no longer worked on its own so I began to incorporate aromatherapy, music, massage and focusing – I had brought a photo of a waterfall for this. I was getting tired and irritated. To give my husband a break I put on a CD by the Beatles with a good 4/4 beat and sang along to it as I swayed, pressing my back against the wall as my contractions came. I sang and sang and sang. As my pain increased (I would describe it as unbearable at this stage) so* did my volume. It had *to, to* match the pain. I needed a change of scenery so I got into the shower and continued singing – I often laughed too, thinking what John, Paul, George and Ringo would have thought! Eventually, I could feel enormous bowel pressure and yelled for the midwife. She examined me and confirmed I was 10 centimetres.

MARTINE *My second birth was more complicated than the first as I had a small bleed from the placenta. This meant I was restricted to bed and monitored throughout the entire labour and I also had an IV inserted into my arm. I found it uncomfortable to use the stress balls that I had used in my first labour, so vocalisation became my main tool. I started, hesitantly, as everyone else on the maternity floor seemed to be fairly quiet. As the pain accelerated so did my voice. At one stage I asked the midwife if the walls in my room were soundproof. 'Don't worry,' she said. 'It is a beautiful sound you are making, it's a musical sound, it's the sound of birthing naturally.' What a wonderful thing to say to me! My husband then said, 'That's right. It's a singing sound, a rhythmic singing sound, keep going.' We are subscribers to the symphony orchestra so I just focused on the beautiful musical sounds I was so used to hearing them perform. The midwife's comments gave me permission to make the sounds and prevented my husband from any embarrassment. I am so grateful to her. I continued confidently until I reached second stage, which involved two pushes and no tear or stitches! Another fabulous birth!*

CELIA *As I hit transition I became overwhelmed by the pain. My 'Aahh' sounds escalated and seemed to naturally progress to 'Ow', 'Ow' (as in 'ouch'). This worked really well for me.*

JODY *During the classes I must admit that I never really raised my voice very much when we had to practise making noise. While I was convinced of the concept of sound blocking pain, I had decided I wanted to get my sound from somewhere else. When we arrived at the hospital, I was 7 centimetres dilated. As labour progressed and the contractions started getting much stronger, my moans turned into long, loud bellows that lasted for the entire contraction. I felt I was using my voice to push the pain out of my body. I remember being shocked at how loud and strong my voice sounded, but it worked. It really helped block the pain, which returned whenever I stopped yelling. So I kept going and kept getting louder and louder. It actually felt really empowering to see how loud I could be and I really didn't care at all that I had turned into a cave woman. We continued like this on and off for about two hours. Throughout I just kept repeating to myself, 'It's just a muscle working,' and 'My baby knows the way.' This stopped me from feeling anxious or scared about what was happening. I kept this up until I reached 10 centimetres and it was time to push. It was exciting to feel such an intense, raw emotion and I almost crave experiencing that intensity again. I was in the moment and it gives me goose bumps to think I actually did it. You know you are doing the biggest most exciting thing you have ever done, and it excites and scares you at the same time. Incredible.*

BELINDA *I kept thinking, 'Focus on the sound,' and this got me through 19 hours of labour.*

ELVA *I began with my yoga breathing but as the pain built up I gradually 'Mmmmmmmed' louder and louder to match the pain. It was a fantastic distraction and, to be honest, I was surprised that it all worked so well.*

JOSIE *After a while the pain was getting really intense so we moved to the shower. I leaned over a plastic chair, the water cascading over my back, and put all my energy into yelling down towards the plug hole. It looked a little like a microphone so I just focused on it until I had the pushing urge.*

JULIE *From the delivery suite window I looked down at a white market umbrella. I would blow out towards each point of that umbrella – around and around and over and over. This technique got me to 5 centimetres, and then I had to bring in more mastery tools.*

ALTHEA *I used my yoga breathing during contractions until I was 5 centimetres dilated, but then I needed more to help me release the tension and pain so I switched to sound. I was still able to use my yoga breathing in between the contractions when there was no pain. This helped me relax my body before the next contraction came.*

NATASHA *As long as I concentrated on the 'Aahh' sound I could not feel when the contraction ended or when the next one began; my husband had to tell me. My husband, with a stopwatch, counted me in three seconds before each one started.*

JAN *I remembered Juju saying that human sound helps release endorphins so I called out loudly each time a contraction came. At first I felt uneasy as it is not something I usually do, but once I got into the rhythm and discovered it actually did block the pain, I had to do it. I was absolutely amazed at the sound I could produce. I didn't know my lungs were capable of such noise – I guess that's part of the adrenalin rush. My husband was amazed as well.*

Remember: **Focus on the sounds of your sounds, not the pain.**

A final thought ...

When I conduct my 'Sound Blocks Pain' session, I spend the second half of the class out in the street. We walk along the footpath of a main road that runs through an area of shops, restaurants and businesses. And we practise.

We practise walking, sitting, leaning, crouching on anything we find along the way.

We practise breathing and vocalising! That's right. In front of everyone.

This is such a worthwhile exercise. Is everyone a little timid to begin with? Yes! Does the group feel embarrassed? Yes! Does the group feel silly? Yes! Does each woman wish she hadn't come to my class that night? Absolutely! But ... do the women find it valuable? Yes! Does the group laugh and talk and start to get courage? Definitely! Does the exercise break down inhibitions? Absolutely! Do the women after the birth say, 'Thank goodness for that class in the street'? All the time!

I saw a short article recently about one of our talented sopranos, Amelia Farrugia. I have enjoyed her performances at the opera for many years and have always admired her voice, her verve and her beauty. I remember her singing 'O Mio Babbino Caro' at an outdoor concert at the Sydney Opera House one year. It was intoxicating! It took my breath away! I was very proud as I had taken a dear friend with me who was a Patron of the Metropolitan Opera House in New York , and he was quite impressed to say the least!

In the article the journalist asked Amelia about whether she utilised her voice in the delivery room during the birth of her first child.

'I'm sure they could hear me three suburbs away. You have an added advantage with a big voice – you can let it all out,' she responded.

Find your voice. Yours can be big too. You may not have a voice for opera, but *everybody* has a voice for birth – adrenalin ensures it! It's a measure of your potential, your authority, your power.

It *is* an incredible human force.
Use it to handle the pain.

You have learnt what to do with the legs, feet and hips. You have added to that the powerful vehicles of breath and sound. Now you need to learn what to do with your eyes in labour; more specifically, during contractions. You never know what you will use to master your pain on the day. Often you will be surprised. The golden rule is: *Be open*. Listen to your contractions. See what they want you to do. You may use just one mastery skill or several. When the pain takes you out of your comfort zone, you may need to detach from it, in every way.

Now you will learn how to do this with your eyes as well.

SKILL # 3

Visualisation

As the members of my class arrive each night throughout the birth skills course I already have a labour visualisation CD playing softly in one section of the room. Sometimes the women are greeting each other and talking so they barely notice the sound; at other times they may close their eyes and follow the script as they sit quietly waiting for each class to begin. So by the time we actually get to the visualisation class they have already done some basic imagery training, whether subliminally or consciously. In this class we build upon that basic skill to diversify and strengthen this extremely valuable technique for childbirth.

I always think of the visualisation class as the most creative session in the course as it involves so many wonderful ways of using the sense of sight, both internal and external. It is not just to help with the skill of relaxation and body awareness, which is important too, but it develops interesting and powerful ways to help manage pain in labour.

When I taught my first antenatal course in the late 1960s visualisation classes did not even exist. I think there was an initial trend to ask the woman to look at a spot on the ceiling (everyone was lying on their backs then, remember) during the contractions. But over the years this one distraction technique expanded to include eye-to-eye contact with partners, blowing at imaginary candles, closing the eyes and centring inwards, and using simple imagery to self-induce a more relaxed state. That's pretty much how it stayed for the next few decades. I still teach those basic visualisation skills today but I also expose the women to far more interesting and dynamic techniques and tools of visualisation so that they can use them more creatively and therefore more effectively on the day of labour.

I arrive at my visualisation class laden with oranges, lemons, sprigs of fresh lavender, contraction charts, colour diagrams of the uterus and cervix, essential oils, photographs of the Sydney Harbour Bridge, dolls, a knitted uterus (imagine that for your first imagery lesson!), cardboard rings to represent the various diameters of dilation of the cervix, coloured ice-lolly sticks marked off in 1-centimetre distances, numbered bathroom tiles, candles, coloured plastic flowers, coloured balls, newspaper billboard sheets, diagrams of the brain and pituitary gland, all sorts of music CDs from bird sounds in Lamington National Park to New Age chimes, panpipes and Mozart, as well as bags and bags of other visual tools to practise with and develop ideas from. This is the one class that never finishes on time!

So you can see, from an original base of the very simple 'focus on a spot' during labour the scope of visualisation and imagery has developed and expanded over the years to encourage women to recruit the sense of sight (internal and external) as a powerful, individual and creative aid to ease labour pain and to facilitate the birth process. In this chapter you are going to learn some of the visualisation techniques that I've found to be the most popular with the couples in my classes. These are the ones they learn and apply so effectively to their labours.

What does visualisation involve?

Visualisation is quite simply the creative faculty or process of forming visual images or ideas, realities, imaginings, scenes, memories, future events, objects, etc., in your mind. During labour, you can use it to help distract you from the pain, reinforce what is happening in your body, and keep you calm. Let's think about it another way. It involves using your eyes as a feedback device to give you specific information; information that you will concentrate on to the exclusion of everything else. You will be using your mind as a huge visual display unit to relay pictures that you can focus on each time a contraction comes. They may be still or moving pictures, coloured or black and white, big or small, related to labour or quite removed from it. Let me stress again, you will be focusing on these so that you do not focus on the pain.

You can have your eyes open (as you would if focusing on a ceiling spot or your partner's eyes) or you can have your eyes closed (as you would if you were using an image in your mind). Let me take you back to your school days for a moment.

Did you ever sit in the playground or laze on the school lawn and dream about the summer holidays? I certainly did – usually just before exam time as I recall! If you lived on the coast, or holidayed abroad, you would probably see in your mind's eye the sun and the surf, and you could not only see the sand under your feet but you could feel it too. You might also see the lifesaver's enclosure and the orange and yellow flags flapping in the wind. Then perhaps your new swimsuit, trendy sunglasses, a colourful towel slung over your shoulder. You may even see a new surfboard, the colour and design of it, the shape of it and, yes, you can definitely see it and feel it as you paddle out to where the best waves start. You can smell the board wax. You are aware of the rise and fall of the waves and the general swell of the ocean beyond. Perhaps, if your holiday was really exotic, you can even see the same porpoises that played in the deep water when you were there last year. And then see yourself catch the perfect wave that takes you into shore. Now you turn around and paddle out once again. You feel so strong, so healthy, and so fully alive! You can see and feel it all. You are right there! Well, almost ...

Oops, there's the school bell, wake up! Back to reality. You leave that beach scene, finish what you are eating, hear your friends talking and laughing, stretch and think about getting back to the classroom where you will be looking at the blackboard and some books and maps for much of the afternoon. The holidays will come, but you have to finish the term and get through the exams first. But, oh, isn't daydreaming wonderful?

Daydreaming is a simple visualisation, and the ways you use the different visual techniques in labour are not too different to imagining the summer holidays or looking at the blackboard or a TV screen in the classroom. Some of the images in this daydreaming exercise were memories, scenes in the future, present, static, moving, colour, black and white, eyes opened, eyes closed, connected to sensation, to sound, to smell, internal screens, external screens, etc. Labour will be less like luxurious daydreaming, though; more like determined concentration, simply due to the presence of the pain. As the pain becomes more intense you will focus on your chosen image with the exquisite intensity of a laser. In fact, the women who had the expectation of beautiful, romantic daydreaming visualisation in labour are the ones who say it didn't work. Using visualisation does not mean you won't be working hard.

KATE *My husband was very creative with a diving analogy – we had done lots of this together. As the contraction came, I closed my eyes as he described the sparkling water and the colourful fish life – the mouthpiece for the gas [nitrous oxide] was a little like a diving mask. His stories were my main skills for the whole of the first stage of labour. He talked and I visualised for seven hours a fantastically positive, encouraging and familiar journey. The poor man got no break – if he paused he got into big trouble from me. He was incredible. I recommend you just pick something you are both familiar with and go on a wonderful, colourful and detailed journey. It was quite amazing how it worked.*

Let's clarify some of the different ways you can recruit your sense of sight to help you in labour, by moving your attention away from the pain. As well as following these ideas, research some of your own. With your eyes open, focus on:

- a spot on the wall, a logo on clothing
- a photograph, a favourite object
- words that are written or printed on objects
- a pattern on furniture, wallpaper, curtain
- your partner's eyes, shirt, watch
- colours, shapes or lights in the room.

These types of images can be big or small, familiar or unfamiliar. You can use either your central or peripheral vision for the above techniques. You can also focus on:

- active images, e.g. crossing a bridge, scuba diving, walking
- watching activities, such as banging stress balls
- bubbles in the spa bath
- blowing at a plastic bottle top floating on the water as you kneel in the bath
- blowing at a candle
- your own reflection in the mirror, tap, shower fixtures
- blowing at a plastic flower floating in the sink.

With your eyes closed, focus on:

- picturing your cervix as it dilates to 10 centimetres
- picturing the baby moving deeper into your pelvis
- picturing the baby rotating in your pelvis.

You can add more emotional intensity to visualising the three activities above by 'willing' them to happen and impressing upon them their ability to happen. But note, although these three activities form the fundamentals of the first stage of labour, you cannot feel them, so you may need your partner to coach you with the keywords 'Open', 'Down', 'Turn', to help you maintain your focus as you do them.

Other images to think about can include:

- focusing on words or numbers in your head
- visualising the pain as waves and swells of energy to help labour progress

- visualising the letting go of muscular tension through your body, sound and breath – 'relax shoulders', 'pain out, panic out', 'breathe and release'
- visualising your vaginal outlet soft and relaxed.

LYNN *In early labour I visualised a period-like pain and imagined it effacing the cervix and beginning to open it up. My husband had bought a wonderful bouquet of flowers to show his love and I focused on these later on. He also led me in 'blowing out the candle' visualisations. I could also see your [Juju's] face saying, 'Healthy pain.' All of these tools helped block the pain.*

There are no rules

Visualisation is very individual and may be used as a primary or secondary birth tool. Here are some guidelines of when to use the techniques in labour, but feel free to change them all around to a way that suits you best. The most important thing to remember about labour is that different techniques suit different women, and all at different times, and just as with all the other skills, you may not use much visualisation at all or you may use it as your main skill.

From 0 to 3 centimetres you could try simple images of ripples and waves of energy and activity across your abdomen, see words that facilitate relaxation, use breathing imagery, blow towards a candle, imagine the musical instruments in the music you are listening to.

From 4 to 7 centimetres you will be working harder to distract from the pain so you or your partner might see and say your favourite keywords, fix your gaze on a power point, imagine the activity your partner is talking you through, look at the plastic stickers or numbers you have attached to the tiles in the shower (make sure they are removable). You will be concentrating hard with the labour process: visualise 'Cervix open', 'Baby down', 'Baby turn'.

From 7 to 10 centimetres it is possible to focus on the internal labour activity, but because it is in the same area as the pain this may take massive amounts of concentration as distraction may be difficult, especially if visualisation is being used as a single technique. Because the pain is so great at this time distraction can be more effective if your attention is somewhere other than near the uterus, so use any of the suggestions listed above. Most women at this stage are using two, three, four or five pain-relieving birth skills at once, so if you have been using visualisation successfully up until this point and it is starting to wane, combine it with some other more powerful techniques at the same time, e.g. stepping, rocking, vocalising, stress balls, and focus on these.

Pushing during second stage labour will usually involve just that – pushing. Every bit of concentration you have will be directed into bearing down and usually your doctor and midwife will encourage this. Your imagery will involve pushing with the correct muscles in the right direction. (See Skill # 6 for more details.)

Crowning will be different for everyone so again the imagery will be variable. Please be aware that if the vaginal outlet is stinging or burning sometimes the last thing on your mind is imagery or visualisation or using a mirror. If you have any spare energy during crowning try to visualise the outlet as soft, relaxed, able to expand, yielding to your baby. You may open your eyes and watch the crowning in a mirror, or, and don't be alarmed, you might just be telling your doctor or midwife to 'get it out!' Finally, your partner may play the most important role here and tell you repeatedly to look into his eyes and pant. (See Skill # 7 for more details.)

Now you have many ideas to consider when using visualisation. In one of my visualisation classes my colleague, aromatherapist Fiona Fanner, joins us to enhance the group's learning about visualisation and oils, and as a tactile addition for extra distraction, we incorporate the fruit and flowers, simply to hold and focus on. We find in labour that the sense of smell is aided by imagery and imagery is enhanced by the sense of smell, and also the sense of touch. We use the billboard notices to visually explore activities, ideas and journeys as well as encouraging stories from the group that we can use creatively. I also bring in a whole lot of ice-lolly sticks (the length of an ice-lolly stick is about 10 centimetres) with one to ten marked along the length of them.

As we move through the imagery exercises for labour, I ask the women to mark off with their thumbs on the ice-lolly sticks, centimetre by centimetre, the dilation of the cervix. The actual image of the measurement helps them to have a realistic idea of the amount their cervix has dilated as their labour proceeds. I also encourage the women to take their stick into labour with them so that, as the midwife examines them, they have an external reference point for dilation. In terms of dilation, they can see where they are and how far they have to go.

I must confess I do have some women who think the topic of visualisation is a little new age and lightweight, but by the time they finish the class their attitude changes significantly. This is because one of the greatest fears women have about labour is the fear of the pain. The fear is made even more difficult on the day as the pain does not even seem to be connected to the labour process. It is, of course, but because you have no sensation of the dilation, rotation, descent processes due to lack of sensory nerves in the area, your anxiety can increase. Labour would be a lot easier if every time you felt the pain you could actually feel a little bit of dilation, rotation and descent. Women would know exactly why the pain was there and be able to relate to it more easily. This is why visualisation can be so powerful. It keeps you connected to something that might otherwise seem meaningless.

WENDY *On the way to the hospital, I banged my stress balls together and focused on one of the colours of the balls, trying to keep my eyes fixed on the colour as I banged. When we arrived at the hospital I focused on a large marble statue of a mother and a baby. In established labour I occasionally looked at a pair of baby's booties to remind me why I was there.*

So each time you have a contraction you will know that the uterus is contracting, the baby is moving down, the baby is turning around. If you understand this and visualise this it will suddenly have meaning for you. If it has meaning, it will inspire you and give you purpose to keep moving forwards. If it inspires you, you can truly own it even though it hurts. This powerful awareness will help block the fear and panic, and with all of this working for you rather than against you, you are halfway there.

Concentrating on what is happening, visualising it in your mind's eye, or disconnecting and distracting from it altogether, will help you focus on only what needs to be done for each contraction. When using visualisation on its own or with other tools or techniques, you need to concentrate on your chosen focus to the exclusion of everything else. Focus like a laser and concentrate exclusively on this.

A little physiology ...

Vision is very important to human functioning; one-third of the brain is devoted to it. The brain has evolved to absorb visual stories easily as it is vital to have pictures and stories to assist us with the development of our memory. In labour, recalling scenes such as walking through a field of lavender or scuba diving around a coral reef shows the power of the mind. Some women even like to visualise their birth physiology during labour, such as adrenalin being depleted or oxytocin flowing or endorphins being released to assist them in the task.

Your eyes send information to the primary visual cortex in your brain. Here, specialised brain cells deal with different aspects of vision, sorting and sending information to other areas for further processing. For example, there is an area of your brain for colour vision and another for visual motion. For complicated sensations like vision, components such as colour, movement, shape and size can be put together so you can see a single object possessing all these properties. It is possible to selectively pay attention to just one of these components, excluding the others, and this comes in useful when mastering labour pain.

FIONA *I was 8 centimetres dilated by the time I got to hospital with my second baby, so labour was well and truly established. I went into the shower and leaned over a plastic chair and started staring at the perforations in the seat, counting them inside my head like an internal chant. I remember distinctly that there were two rows of three holes and one row of four holes separating them, and I counted them over and over again. I don't think I'll ever forget that pattern as long as I live. It was absolutely the most important thing in the world to me at the time. Soon I was into second stage and after about four pushes my baby was born. As you [Juju] mentioned in one of your classes, the cup of tea the midwife brought in after it was all over was the best cup of tea I've ever drunk, or will ever drink!*

If you pick up stress balls, you know the balls have colours, size and shape, even if they are moving fast, such as when you are banging them together. If you focus on the rhythm of the movement of your arms as you move them in and out of your central and peripheral vision, the colour, size and shape become secondary; the movement becomes your primary focus. On the other hand, you may focus on the colour, or you could even use your ears to focus on the sound of the balls hitting each other as your primary focus. Concentrating on one aspect of the balls pushes all the other details into the background, including the pain.

Putting it into practice

If visualisation is your main labour skill you will need an environment that supports this. It is difficult to accomplish with a lot of chatter around, for instance. As your contractions sweep through your body you will need to raise the intensity of your concentration to enable you to focus on the imagery and not the pain. Never fear, though: your friendly fight/flight reflex will give you the advantage of being able to focus your mind more acutely when you are in pain than when you are not.

Detach yourself from 'looking' at the pain by visualising something else. Isolate something to focus on – keep it simple, nothing is right or wrong – and concentrate on this exclusively with your eyes open or closed. When you find your chosen image, focus with the intensity of a laser until the 60 seconds are over, then rest.

In the last trimester of pregnancy, start to change any negative messages you may have about labour. For example, you might visualise yourself losing control – change that to an image of yourself working and moving and breathing and focusing. You may be influenced by friends saying things like, 'Just go for the drugs' – think to yourself, 'Yes, that's one option, but I may try some of my own techniques first.' You may be asking yourself, 'How can I cope with the pain?' I hope you can almost write a book on it yourself by the time you finish this one!

All of this dialogue is normal, but turn your focus to strong positive images of yourself releasing, emptying, pushing, opening and greeting your baby. In labour, losing control expends an enormous amount of energy. If you are going to use all of that, try to use it usefully. Have a look at 'Your action plan' (see the next page) and add your own thoughts to it. There is no right way to do this: just do what works for you.

Visualisation exercises

Visualisation works consciously and unconsciously, so practise these techniques as often as you can – even if it is just for a few minutes a day. Some of the positions you might try them in include standing, sitting, kneeling, all fours, leaning over the kitchen bench or kitchen sink, in the shower, the bath and when walking with your partner. You can practise the exercises in a reclining position, with your eyes closed, listening to some soft music, with the phone and television turned off. Ask your partner to read the scripts to you sometimes. I also want you to practise them standing upright and moving with your eyes open, also with more rhythmic music, with your partner by your side. You don't know what position you will adopt on the day, so the more variations to your practice the better you can prepare for the birth.

If your attention easily strays, don't worry, this is normal, just keep bringing it back to your scripted focus. This, of course, will happen in labour as well, and your partner will bring you back to your chosen focus – this is why the practice is good for your partner too.

Your action plan

- Work at rhythmically releasing, e.g. breathing, swaying and visualising a calm expression on your face.
- Work with your own empowering images, e.g. cervix opening, baby moving down, powerful action and purposeful pain.
- Work with your own physiology as you know what is happening – visualise your oxytocin releasing, your adrenalin depleting, your endorphins mobilising even if you are just visualising the words in your head.
- Work with any visual project that helps you master your pain – make a list now, perhaps using the women's labour stories throughout the book for ideas.
- Work at it deliberately – this will take energy, but when you use your mind's eye deliberately, you will not be so focused on the pain.
- Use your energy constructively to focus on positive action and not on negative messages.

IMAGINING THE UNSEEN

Sit quietly, with some soft music playing in the background. Close your eyes. Relax. When you are ready, think about the inside of your body. Visualise your baby, uterus, umbilical cord, amniotic fluid and cervix. Focus on this image in your mind's eye. Then use concentration enhancement to zoom in on your cervix. Watch it open. Breathe it open. Focus on your baby, visualise her head. Watch your uterus; see it as it will be in labour. See it contracting. See it squeezing your baby's head down, down, down into your pelvis, down on to your soft dilating cervix, stimulating the opening of the cervix even more. **Focus like a laser and concentrate exclusively on this**.

Note: After finishing this exercise during pregnancy, be sure to visualise your cervix tightly closed.

WALKING TOGETHER

Lie down on your bed with your partner beside you, and with soft music playing in the background. Close your eyes while he takes you on an imaginative walk up and down the streets near your home. He needs to talk to you for periods of 60 seconds, then rest and be quiet for 30 seconds, then continue on the walk again. Listen to him as he guides you, for example: 'Go out our front door and see our gate and fence. Walk out to the footpath and look up at the sky. What is the weather like today? Then walk across to the other side of the street. How wide is the road? Is there traffic? Keep walking. Now rest for 30 seconds.' Thirty seconds later he continues the walk, describing the houses or apartments of your neighbourhood that you know well, the gardens perhaps. Keep visualising all this in your mind. He could ask you questions: 'Do you see any cars, buses, trams, trucks? Do you see any people, park benches? Do you see any animals? Keep walking. Now rest for 30 seconds.' Continue this journey until you come back to your own front door again. **Focus like a laser and concentrate exclusively on this**.

Add another step: Vary your walks. Try places other than in your neighbourhood, maybe somewhere further away, perhaps where you went on a holiday.

Add another step: Progress to practising this visualisation while you are upright and walking on the spot, which is how you might be at your birth.

FLOWER POWER

Play some beautiful music, relax and close your eyes. Focus on your breathing then imagine you are visiting a flower shop. Look at all the flowers around you, see all the colours. Breathe in the fragrances. Then focus your attention on just one flower; name that flower in your mind. Say it over and over, slowly, in your head. Feel the joy these flowers bring you. Feel soft, and relaxed, and peaceful while you look at them. Look closely at the petals, and imagine them when they were only a young bud on your flower ... then watch them open ... see them blooming ... look at them wilting ... watch them dropping gently to the floor. Reach out and pick them up, feel them, like velvet in the palm of your hand. Blow gently at them, focus on your breathing. Blow gently again, focus on the colours of the wilted petals, the faded fragrance, the softness, the lightness. Focus on your breathing again. Relax.

Add another step: Smell the actual flower if you have it, or the essential oil of that flower on a tissue.

Focus like a laser and concentrate exclusively on this.

Note: Maybe take a few of your favourite flowers with you to inspire this visualisation.

COLOUR BEATS

Pick up your stress balls. Tap them together. Bang them together. Breathe in rhythm with your stress ball activity. Keep everything synchronised and rhythmic. As you work with them, notice their colours. Now notice the colours of your stress balls out of your peripheral vision (the vision at the sides of your eyes). Focus on the colours only with your peripheral vision. Do you see red? Blue? Keep doing this for 60 seconds, the time of your contraction. **Focus like a laser and concentrate exclusively on this**.

WATERFALL

Close your eyes and imagine you are in labour. You are in the shower and the water is falling softly on your abdomen and back. Feel it. Relax. Stay calm. You are standing, but you feel like a rag doll or like a flag that hangs limply when no wind blows. Release any tension. Let the pain go. Visualise the water washing away your pain, your stress. As your contraction builds, start swaying. Let the movement help to release more stress. Visualise the water, the movement. Move, sway, feel the water, let it wash away the pain. Keep your breath rhythmic. Breathe and sway, and breathe and sway, and feel the water. It is washing away the pain. Washing away the stress. It's helping, it's washing the pain away ... keep breathing, keep visualising.

Add another step: Practise this while you shower.

Focus like a laser and concentrate exclusively on this.

SIGHTS AND SOUND

Visualise yourself in labour. See yourself breathing and blowing, and moving and focusing. Watch your breath, slow, long, releasing, relaxing. See yourself vocalising and swaying and focusing. Watch yourself making the sound. Focus only on the sound you are making. See yourself from the inside, making the 'Aahh' sound. It travels out of your body, taking the pain and stress with it. You are in control, your sound giving you much of that command. Listen to the sound you are making. Focus on this sound. Visualise yourself, strong, working, in command, until 60 seconds has passed. **Focus like a laser and concentrate exclusively on this**.

FRAGRANT BUBBLES

Visualise yourself kneeling in the spa bath, if you have one, during labour. The spa jets are on, bubbles surround you, and you are leaning forwards on to a soap rack placed across the bath with a plastic pillow on top of the rack. Smell your favourite essential oil on a tissue. If it is lavender, visualise the flower. If it is citrus, visualise the fruit. For the first half of a contraction, keep vocalising and visualising the lavender or fruit. For the second half, blow the bubbles away. Use your breath to blow a pathway through the bubbles in the spa. Watch the bubbles move. Keep blowing. Focus on blowing a pathway through the bubbles for 30 seconds, until the contraction has gone. **Focus like a laser and concentrate exclusively on this**.

Note: You might want to take some sponge pads to cushion your knees for when you are in the spa bath during labour.

BLOWING OUT THE CANDLE

Light a candle in your mind. See the candle then focus on the flame. Look at the colour of the candle, then the flame. Breathe towards the candle, slowly then quickly to work out which is the right speed for you at this time. Smell the fragrance of the candle. Breathe and blow. Watch and visualise. Smell and relax. Release the pain, relax the stress, visualise the candle, blowing the flame, until the 60 seconds is complete.

Add another step: See the candle in different places – close up, far away, on the window sill, on the bedside table. Picture your labour room – the room may be dark with just the flame of the candle giving light, or bright and the candle is unlit. **Focus like a laser and concentrate exclusively on this**.

Note: I encourage class members to fix a feather on to a candle wick to help with this visualisation as hospital policy usually prevents a lighted flame in the delivery suite. Also the fragrant wax can sometimes cause nose irritation for some women. Check this out long before the day.

COUNT UP, COUNT DOWN

As your partner counts, see the numbers in your mind's eye. Listen to the counting, the numbers. Visualise them. See a **1** (or a one, spelt out). See a **2**. See a **3**. See a **4**. See a **5**. See a **6**. Hear your partner counting these numbers but look at the numbers. Breathe in time with the counting. Count out loud and hear your voice but see the numbers. See the numbers being drawn on a blackboard in your mind. Focus on hearing and seeing the numbers, until 60 seconds are up. **Focus like a laser and concentrate exclusively on this**.

TURN ON THE TAP

Play some soft music and let your mind drift. Allow your attention to flow with the melody. Then bring your attention to the process of your labour. Focus on the brain chemicals involved. Imagine oxytocin as a pink colour and watch it flow from your brain into your bloodstream and into your uterine muscle. Visualise a tap that allows this hormone to flow or to shut down. Visualise the tap is turned on – stress can turn the tap off so see yourself releasing that stress so the tap stays on. See the oxytocin flowing freely. See your uterus contracting. Keep releasing the stress and keep that tap turned on. Watch the pink fluid flowing freely. **Focus like a laser and concentrate exclusively on this**.

Partner's role

- Take your cue from her:
  - sometimes it helps more to stand back, be quiet, to watch and wait
  - sometimes it helps to talk rhythmically, e.g. 'Red, red, red', as she stares at the red colours of the stress balls.
- Have a list of her preferred visualisations and remind her of the variety of images available for her (read the bullet points in the previous 'What does visualisation involve?' section again and the women's labour reports for lots of great suggestions).
- If visualisation is too passive, lead her to a more active pain mastery skill.
- Add physical visual reminders of the visualisations, such as small number or flower stickers (newsagents have them) to the tiles in the shower, to assist the visualisation.
- Be respectful of hospital policies and don't light a candle if not permitted, and remove any images, such as the numbers, when you leave the delivery suite.

And now over to Sarah. I must admit, I didn't know my raggedy old doll, which incidentally is called William, made such an impression on her, but I'll let her tell you about it.

Sarah's story

My third class. I was now looking forward to coming and as I entered the room I sat down with a few of the other mums-to-be like an old hand, not the new girl any more. Juju was sticking up large posters along the wall. She'd pinned up three pictures that together made up one of our most recognisable icons, the Sydney Harbour Bridge; they were, in sequence, the southernmost end, the middle of the bridge, and the northernmost end. She also had three pictures of a woman's pelvis: the first showed a baby pushing on the cervix, in the second the baby was pushing through the cervix, and the third showed the baby making its way out through the vagina.

This class was about how visualisation can be an important tool in mastering labour pain. Juju was creating for us constructive images to focus on to distract us from the pain. The images would also help us to stay focused on what our bodies were doing through each contraction. Initially I didn't quite understand how the bridge would do that but I could see how thinking about and knowing how the uterus was working – contracting in order to push the baby further down the pelvis and onto the cervix, encouraging it to dilate and open – would.

It wasn't long before Juju had us standing up, moving and vocalising as usual, but this time she gave us an image to think about as well. This is where the bridge came in. We had to imagine we were at the start of a contraction and then turn our focus onto the southern pylon of the bridge, the beginning of our 'walk'. We then visualised walking up the arc of the bridge, just like the bridge climbers do, as the contraction progressed. Halfway through the contraction we reached the middle of the bridge. Then we walked down the other side for the second half of the contraction. 'Almost there,' Juju said, before we reached the northernmost end, the finish. As we got to the end of the climb in our minds, we also came to the end of our imagined 60-

second contraction. By visualising something familiar and being able to see an end, the end of the walk, helped us to stay remarkably focused on the positive, which in this case was the passing of time till the end of the contraction. I've since learnt that the power of the imagination to change our mental state, especially when in excruciating pain, is an incredible skill.

NICOLE *After I got into the spa I got up on to my knees and stared intensely at a label on a towel on the edge of the bathtub. It said, 'Spotless Linen.' I read it over and over. I will never forget those two words. Later, I stared at the white button on my husband's polo shirt.*

I used visualisation throughout my labour. I thought about using the types of journeys like the bridge climb, but for me the most effective was focusing on my baby's journey – what was actually happening to me physically during my labour. I recalled Juju's pictures of the baby – first high up in the pelvis, then pushing through the pelvis and the cervix, and finally out the vagina – and recalled them to help me. Juju also used objects to give us even more concrete images for this visualisation. She had a doll, which she used as a baby, and a plastic pelvis. As she explained the physicality of labour she rotated the baby to illustrate how it turns down towards the cervix, then pushed the baby through the pelvis and out. Repeatedly. Every 10 minutes or so in class Juju would show us the baby moving down towards its birth. While this constant repetition at the time seemed unnecessary, the result was that I certainly had very strong visual images to take with me into the delivery suite.

One of the most invaluable lessons I learnt from Juju's classes was what was actually happening to my body and to my baby during labour. I can't stress how much this changed my focus from one of fear and uncertainty to absolute confidence and control. Juju showed us how the uterine muscle works to bring the baby towards its birth. We also learnt that this pain – healthy pain – is due to the fatigue of the uterine muscle working, not the actual uterus hurting. The pain can also be referred to other areas of your body, which is why some women have the pain in the tummy, some down their thighs. Juju describes the pain you feel during labour as 'only a muscle working'. I can't tell you how many times in my labour I reminded myself of this: 'It is only a muscle working.' It became a kind of mantra for me (see Skill # 5).

What all this information meant for me was that when my obstetrician, Keith, told me how dilated I was I understood exactly what stage I was at and where the baby was. I can only encourage you to have an appreciation of the mechanics of labour by the time your contractions arrive. It does help. Because labour is long and so extremely painful I found I often forgot what I was doing there! The strenuous physicality of labour began to overtake my mental state. I would lose sight of what I was working so hard for – the birth of my baby – but by visualising my uterus working, and working hard to open my cervix and bring my baby down, I brought my focus back to why I was actually there. It was this visualisation that helped me stay positive throughout my labour. I could see the uterine muscle working in my mind. I could see it contracting. I knew it was working hard, bringing my baby into the world.

HELEN *My husband would say to me, 'Visualise your cervix opening.' After a vaginal examination confirmed 3 centimetres of dilation, he would say, 'Imagine it opening to 4 centimetres,' then 'Imagine it opening to 5 – come on, you can do this, imagine 5, we are pushing for 5.' Maybe this was a man's way of saying things, but at the next examination, an hour later, I was 5.5 centimetres. My husband was amazed and I was over the moon.*

Juju always repeated to us, 'See the baby moving down, pushing down, opening the cervix, pushing, pushing. Open and down. Open and down. Down and out. Down and out. Come on baby. Down and out. Bring the baby down.' Her words were with me, and as my contractions increased I almost cheered them on: 'Come on. Work on opening the cervix.' I could see what my baby was doing. Pushing his head down. Working his way out. This way I also bonded with my baby. We were working through this together. I could see my beautiful baby. And I could see him being born.

It is not only the pain that can make you lose sight of this but the simple fact that you can't feel your cervix. You can't feel it opening. You can't feel the baby working its way down. You have absolutely no sensation of the internal movements or process of birth. This is why being able to visualise them is important. It was good to be able to remind myself that this was healthy pain: my body is doing what it is so supposed to be doing, helping my little miracle into this world. I would immediately feel more positive and have a new surge of beneficial energy. Without seeing Juju's three images of the baby moving through the cervix (and her rag doll and pelvis for extra measure) it wouldn't have been ingrained into my head. I could call upon the images when I needed them. I did need them, and this method really worked for me.

CAMERON *I had planned to time the contractions in labour and tell my wife when she was halfway through the 60 seconds. I really didn't plan it beforehand, but I started to tell her she was mountain biking up a hill. We both do some mountain biking, so she visualised this. When the contraction started I said, 'Okay, here comes the hill.' At 15 seconds I said, 'Come on, keep pedalling, you are halfway up the hill,' or 'You are nearly at the top, keep breathing.' When we got to 30 seconds I said, 'You've reached the top – you're on your way down now.' My wife focused on every word I said.*

Visualisation, on the one hand, is one of the easiest things to do during labour because no one can see you doing it but it's also quite challenging when you are doing it with a contraction and with pain. For me, it was simply a great positive reinforcement. Believe it or not, even though I was focused on movement and sound I still had room in my mind to think about the pain! So, in that extra space I kept the image of my baby's movement down through the pelvis active in my mind. Whether you use visualisation to distract your mind from the pain, to take yourself to another place or, like me, you use it to focus on the birthing process, it is a very powerful tool.

The extraordinary thing about visualisation is the diversity of ways in which it is used by women during labour. As you read the labour excerpts in this chapter you'll notice similarities as well as the differences. Be inspired by them as they worked well for these women and maybe one or some of the ideas will help you.

TEYA   *I was staring at the word 'Hot' on the tap.*

NATASHA   *Initially, I was walking around the house, rolling on the fit ball, concentrating on my baby and willing it to move down, all the time reminding myself that it was good pain. By the time we reached the hospital the contractions were more painful and closer together. I used the stress balls, banging them together at first, concentrating on the blue segments. Everything needed to be blue and my husband helped by pointing out other blue objects for me. My husband's support was so important – I could not bear it if he walked away. As labour became more and more painful, I instinctively pointed at objects – the light switch, ornaments on the wall, or any object in the delivery room – and blew at them. In my mind I was trying to blow air to each object and move it. I could not explain this to my husband or midwife and I'm sure they wondered what on earth I was doing! I found that pointing, watching, blowing and holding the stress balls helped to distract me from the pain.*

ELENA   *I went 14 hours visualising 'baby down' and focusing on the colours of the stress balls until they finally fell apart! In my mind, I turned the pain into the force that was moving my baby deeper and deeper into the pelvis.*

NARELLE *I focused on cue cards propped up against the lounge and I really took on board the words and their meanings.*

ANNIE *I visualised a waterfall we had visited in New Zealand while cool water was sprayed on my face. Later on I used eye contact with my husband as he was counting me through the contractions.*

FELICITY *I would visualise the pain being released through my mouth with my 'Aahh' sound. I had no fear of the pain in doing this technique, although I would have to say it was extremely challenging!*

DENISE *I would picture the classes, I could see your [Juju's] face, I could hear you talking, and those images gave me something to hang on to.*

CELIA *I found it impossible to focus on anything except a spot on the wall and then a flower on the curtain.*

WENDY *As I counted backwards from 100 I could see the numbers clearly in my head. This was all I saw – with my eyes sometimes open and sometimes closed.*

HOLLIE *At the beginning of each contraction, my husband guided me visually down the stairs at our local beach, past the surf club, then on towards the beachside shops, which would culminate with the peak of the contraction. Along the way he would mention the surfers and the waves breaking on the beach. Meanwhile I would have my eyes shut, picturing the whole scene in my head as well as using vocalisation to help me through the pain. As the contraction eased, he guided me further, past the next surf club, a surf swimming pool and finally to our favourite beachside kiosk where we would rest. For variation, he took me on other familiar walks, mentioning landmarks I knew. For me, these techniques were so effective my midwife often had to tell me my contraction was over, as I hadn't realised it myself. I was not focused on the pain at all – I was focused on the walk. My husband was fantastic!*

CATHY *As I bounced gently on a big fit ball I kept visualising, bringing my baby's head gently down on to the cervix. I knew this would make the labour more efficient and it did. At 8 centimetres I changed my internal focus from the baby and cervix and stared outwardly at the logo on my husband's shirt.*

SHONA *The only time I used visualisation was in transition, when I pictured your [Juju's] face and other images from class. I pictured you saying, 'Go,' and I did. Then five contractions later I was fully dilated.*

SALLY *I focused on a picture of a waterfall that I had taken on a holiday. I imagined so much about that waterfall, it's all I needed.*

MELINDA *I found myself focusing on the movement of my arm as I crossed the shower nozzle across my belly.*

KATE *The plug hole in the shower looked like a microphone, so I just focused on this and yelled down it.*

KATIA *I focused on the little red light at the bottom of the television set.*

KATE *During contractions I stared intently out the window and fixed my eyes on three ventilator pipes. When the pain became bigger, I added stress balls, foot stamping and the 'Aahh' sound – all rhythmic and all in time – and just stared at those blessed ventilator pipes!*

CARL *My wife explained the concept of bombarding as many senses as possible during labour to help distract her from the pain and we discussed many options for the visualisation techniques she had learned in classes as we wanted to be as prepared as we could. Before the birth we discussed our memories of hiking in the Rocky Mountains and Tunnel Mountain in Banff as we had done this many times. As it turned out we used a different visualisation on the day. My wife was standing in almost a 'skier's tuck' position during contractions. At the same time she was very hot. Very hot! This gave me the idea to get her to imagine us skiing in minus 30 degrees Celsius weather. I talked her through the contractions, asking her to remember the beautiful soft, white snow whooshing under her skis as she zoomed down the mountain. I asked her to focus on the wind in her face and the crisp air hitting her cheeks. After the birth my wife told me just how helpful this had been. It relieved the heat she was feeling and took her mentally back to that wonderful place. In the most painful part of labour, she found it invigorating and was surprised at how useful it was. She heard every word I said, and used the whole story to escape from the pain.*

KYLIE *My visualisation alternated between watching the pathway of my breath and me lying on a lilo in a swimming pool in Hawaii. I would focus on images in that magical place as my husband timed 15, 30, 45 and 60 seconds for each contraction.*

Remember: **Focus like a laser and concentrate exclusively on this.**

A final thought ...

Now you have some tangible ideas about how you can recruit the use of your mind and eyes in labour. Some of you will find visualisation and concentration enhancement too passive, or for whatever reason it will not be in your skills bag for mastering pain. It may be secondary to something else you are using to stay in command. However, the women who use it say it is brilliant.

Focusing in the first stage of labour is fundamental to control, and matching the pain with your chosen primary birth skill is vital to blocking your brain's perception of pain. So if with your visualisation techniques you need to add other, more physical birth skills, like stress balls or stepping, then explore the introduction of them to see which one best accompanies visualisation. Then if you need to make one of these your primary technique, use visualisation as a secondary technique, or let it go altogether, and then reintroduce it in second stage for pushing and crowning.

The next pain mastery tool is brilliant for blocking pain, working off adrenalin and mobilising large amounts of your endorphins: stress balls.

SKILL # 4

Stress balls

I was two weeks overdue with my daughter, Marina. It was my first birth and, I must say, during the nine and a half months of that pregnancy I did not give the birth much thought at all. When I went into labour I remembered clearly the instructions we'd learnt in our antenatal classes: 'Relax your face ... relax your hands ... relax your body.' As far as practical preparation went, that was it – besides instructing us to breathe. The active birth philosophy did not hit until 1983, and even then it was slow to catch on.

I *thought* it would be easy; all I needed to do was simply follow those instructions and relax my face, relax my hands, relax my body. Even my husband remembered the instructions, telling me to 'Relax your hands. Relax your face. Relax your body ... Come on, just try to relax,' while I was in labour.

This technique of passive relaxation worked for me for a while, but as the pain increased in intensity all it did was induce in me a state in which I was swamped with even more stress. There I was lying on that bed, on my back, consumed by pain! Someone suggested I focus on an image of a wave washing over me but, I can assure you, reclining in pain is no place to think about a wave washing over you. It was just another nail in the coffin, so to speak. I was overwhelmed with pain very quickly and could no longer continue under my own steam. I had an epidural when I was around 2 to 3 centimetres dilated, and then a top-up later on.

I simply had no effective resources to cope as the pain began to accelerate. For me, and I do acknowledge that birth and pain technique preferences are very individual, the gentle tools of breathing and relaxation just didn't do it. And nor did being stuck on that bed! Thank goodness for the introduction a decade later of a more active approach to relaxation and pain management during childbirth.

Active hands block pain

One way of being active during labour or, more specifically, one way of actively relaxing (sounds paradoxical, doesn't it?) so you can decrease both stress and pain, is by using your hands. Forget those limp wrists and put your good, strong hands to work. Activities such as squeezing and banging stress balls can make an incredible difference in how you master your pain. Sounds unorthodox? Maybe, if you have never done it before, but activity with your hands will go much further in blocking your pain, mobilising your endorphins and providing non-painful rhythmic activity for you to focus on when that surge of adrenalin hits you than still, ineffectual hands!

I introduced my first stress ball class in 1989 after one of my class members, Trisha Goddard (at the time on Australian TV's 'The 7.30 Report' and 'Play School', and now, of course, with her own highly successful TV talk show in the UK), rang with her report about the birth of her first child. She had a great birth, working her way through with a combination of tools, particularly loud vocalisation such as the 'Aahh' sound. Interestingly, she also used a rhythmic punching action with her hands throughout the duration of the strong contractions. I did not teach her this in my classes, she just did it spontaneously. And it helped. The combination of loud vocal sounds and the steady beat of her right fist into her left open palm, over and over again until each contraction was finished, seemed to be necessary for Trisha as a pain-management skill. She said it was brilliant and helped her get through her labour without any drugs or an epidural.

As I sat at my desk listening to her story, understanding the physiology behind her hand activity, my mind was running wild with ideas of yet another strategy I could introduce into my classes. I had to work out a way to resemble what Trish was doing; it had to be easy, rhythmic, inexpensive and not too tiring, a dull thump rather than a loud disturbing noise, and acceptable for use in a labour room or delivery suite. In other words, it couldn't be a bongo drum! This is how my stress ball class evolved and this is what this chapter is all about.

A little physiology ...

Under your skin lie the touch sensors: nerves, blood vessels, sweat glands and hair roots. The nerves in this area send information to your spinal cord, which carries the messages to your brain where the sensation is registered. The hands, especially the fingertips, have one of the highest concentrations of touch nerve endings in the body, and they have large areas allocated to register them in the brain. Can you imagine how many burnt fingers we would have from hot kitchen pots and pans if these nerves, and our associated reflexes, were not part of us? If you want to block your brain's perception of pain you can engage your hands and fingers in a pain-free activity that would make an impression on the nerves under the skin, as the messages from this activity would be transported via the spinal cord to the brain and be registered there. You can then consciously focus on these pain-free messages from your hands so that you don't focus on the pain. That is, *focus on the hands, not the pain*.

You will be working with the principle that the brain can only focus on one dominant project at any time. Tapping, squeezing and banging stress balls are an ideal pain-free, rhythmic activity to do with your hands and to focus on. It's so simple.

The hands have always been used by human beings in threat, crisis, emergency or challenging situations – grasping, gripping, pushing, pulling, banging, thumping, striking or even assisting with running, climbing, crouching, etc., or with holding, lifting, swinging and so on.

Our hands help us with our own protection and survival, and some times the protection or survival of another. Using hands is instinctive and is a reflex.

One of the problems with the hands in the childbirth situation is that if you don't know what to do with them they usually clench up with fear and pain and panic. The adrenalin takes over and, if you are unable to accomplish the 'relax your face, relax your hands, relax your body' thing you will find yourself at the beginning of a downward spiral of distress This will give you exactly what you don't want: more pain, more panic more fear. You will start to focus on the pain, which brings even more pain more fear, more panic and more stress. This quickly becomes distress.

Adrenalin needs to be worked off so that it does not impede your labour. Think of the body's adrenalin rush filling your body as a petrol tank being filled up with petrol. The petrol is to make the car go, no stand still with the brakes on! Do not try to go with the brakes on: that won't work either. The adrenalin is the fuel to make your body go, no freeze up in fear.

I have asked you this before (*repetition*, remember): What would adrenalin say if it could talk? That's right, it would say, 'Do something Go! Get up! Move! Brakes off! Put your foot on it!' When the adrenalin rushes in, energy is provided – just in case you need it for protection o survival – but it has nowhere to go. So try working it off with your hands and don't forget to focus on that work to get your mind off the pain.

KIM *On arrival at hospital I was 4 centimetres dilated. I tried lying on the floor mattress, some massage and the fit ball, but I just could not stay still. I got up, paced around my room – the more intense the pain, the faster I paced. Then I needed something extra so I started to use the stress balls. Pacing and banging, pacing and banging, and occasion ally incorporating an 'Aahh' here and there. I did not care which colour were hitting together, but I did need to count, in my head, from one t eight, over and over, with the pacing and the banging for the duration of each 60-second contraction. Pacing and banging and counting, pacing and banging and counting.*

What do you actually do with them?

Stress balls must be of soft resistance, not hard like tennis balls, not soft like foam, and ideally be coloured for extra visual focus. Begin by rhythmically squeezing and releasing one ball as a contraction begins. Focus on what you are doing with your hand. Continue squeezing and releasing with the rate and rhythm that best suits you and your early labour pain. Squeeze and release with the rate and repetition that best matches the level of pain in the contraction. Keep squeezing and releasing for the duration of the contraction, then stop and rest the hand.

Progress to squeezing and releasing two stress balls simultaneously and increase the rhythm, rate of repetition and strength of the grip as the pain increases. *Focus on the stress balls, not the pain.* Create a pattern of doing this throughout each contraction until it ends. Continue using stress balls as long as they are helping or rest for a while and return to them later and add extra pain birth skills as you need them. When squeezing is no longer adequate to help distract you from the pain begin lightly tapping the balls together and then progress to banging them in rhythm with your breath, voice or foot movements.

Keep your hands busy so that they are not just hanging there waiting to clench up with the pain. Experiment with everything. You may just need a soft, gentle activity with your hands, perhaps rubbing them together slowly or rubbing fabric, or you may need to bang those stress balls on the wall. Tap into the potential of all the techniques available at will. Whatever works best for you.

TEYA *The car trip to the hospital was excruciating. I could never have coped without the stress balls. During each contraction I banged them together as hard as I could. I had to have the yellow sides together and as I banged I chanted 'Aahh', 'Aahh', 'Aahh'. On admission at the maternity unit, the midwife said I was in transition.*

What's your objective here?

You need to overload your sensory systems with non-painful stimuli to override the uterine pain signal in the brain. Your brain should register the stress ball activity and not the pain. Just try it. As labour progresses and the pain intensifies start to think 'kettle drums', 'cymbals', 'baseball mitt', 'hammer', and go for it! I've said before, whatever it takes. Of course, avoid all hand movements if they are not right for you.

Labour pain is healthy pain and you can have a healthy response to it. Sick pain – think migraine, endometriosis, infection, gastritis, etc. – is unhealthy pain and it is quite normal to cringe, clench, cry, close down and moan. One creates energy, the other zaps it. Use your stress balls to create a healthy response to your healthy pain. The more intense the pain, the more intense your ball banging becomes.

At the beginning of the stress ball class I show the women some of the different hand tools my past class members have used during labour and then donated to my collection afterwards, along with their tales about how they went. These tools include corporate stress figures, bubble wrap, amethyst rocks, squeezy penguins, rubber boxing kangaroos, big balls, small balls, balls with lights in them, balls with bells on them, and much more. We all have a laugh and admire their ingenuity.

I then read out some of the labour reports. The women describe in detail how these tools were used to block pain and we analyse the details. What exactly did they do with these tools? How did they block the pain? How did they help them with fear and panic? What did their husbands do to help? What other techniques did they recruit to add extra distraction? As a teacher, I always find it fascinating to help the group learn about the methods of others. We also watch a birth DVD of a woman banging her way through her pain in labour with stress balls, and the women in the class always watch with fascination.

At first, the class members are a little sceptical, and rightly so as usually not one woman in the room, except my past clients, has ever used such simple activities to deal with enormous stress. So the inhibition level is understandably high. I am always aware that with teaching the stress ball class to the women there is a fine line between them feeling silly and gaining the confidence to equip themselves with a very simple yet power-ful pain-, stress- and panic-relieving technique for labour. Feelings of embarrassment are always discussed and legitimised, and again, the physiology is explained. Without the physiological reasoning behind the skill, it may not be understood or attempted on the day.

If you feel a little embarrassed during labour, close the door for privacy, play some music to mask your sounds, and ask your partner to count for you to help you keep a beat. I can assure you, if it helps your pain you will get into such a rhythm you won't even notice anyone around you, let alone care who might be watching or what they are thinking. Mostly women worry unnecessarily: the midwives are always brilliant about these methods!

Think of it another way. Take something simple (a rhythmic squeez-ing or banging) and use it to your advantage by taking it to a superior level when you need to match the pain more. Focus on it so hard that this focus supersedes all other awareness.

Not one of my couples goes into labour without their stress balls! Well, that's not really true. One of my class members, Carol, went into labour early and she arrived at the hospital without her stress balls. No problem. She instructed her husband to remove his socks, bundle them up as though they were back in the drawer at home, and used them as 'stress socks' instead. For the next two births she had those stress balls packed!

These activities may seem way out and even ridiculous, but they were incredibly significant for the women who used them as you will read in some of their stories later. Significant, that is, in helping distract them from the pain.

Working with stress balls in different positions

- Standing up: squeezing or banging them together.
- Sitting down: squeezing or banging together or rub or roll on your thighs.
- On your hands and knees: banging on the mattress or floor.
- Lying on your side: squeezing in hands or banging on the side of the bed or rubbing on your upper thigh.
- Support squatting: squeezing in hands.
- In the shower: banging together or on the wall tiles.
- On a fit ball: squeezing or banging together or rubbing on your thighs.
- In the spa bath: squeezing or banging them together or banging on the side of the bath.

Stress ball skills

Practise the following mastery techniques, putting your own stamp on them as you wish. You can use music to help you with a beat and remember, if you feel a little uncomfortable at first it will get easier. I have women who tell me after this class that they will *never* use stress balls in labour, yet they are the same ones who report back to me that they were the main tools to help them block the pain.

I really do encourage you to reserve your judgement regarding stress balls, and I urge you to pack them in your labour kit bag whether you think you will use them or not. As I say to the women in my classes, there is no way I would spend such precious time in my course on this technique if it was not valuable. Practise with them before labour and give them a trial run at home and in the car at the beginning of labour so that you can get used to them.

The following exercises are designed to help you explore the different ways the stress ball activities can help you in labour. You might be banging the stress balls, yet be focused on the colours, or the rhythm, or the shape, or the sound. The most important thing to remember is that, as you use your stress balls, you must focus on them with your eyes, your ears, your thoughts, etc. – do not focus on the pain.

COLOUR AWARENESS

As you bang the balls together focus on the individual colours. Use your central vision first, staring straight at them, then use your peripheral vision, watching them out of the corners of your eyes, and looking past them.

Add another step: Move your feet while you blow towards the balls, and then blow just past them, or even try blowing up towards the ceiling. **Focus on the balls, not the pain**.

Note: Did you know that during your fight/flight response the pupils in your eyes widen to let in more light and improve your peripheral vision? This enables you to see better in the dark, especially at night, and also to focus well in labour.

LISTEN CLOSELY

As you bang the balls together focus on the sound of the bang. At the same time, slowly sway your hips from side to side. **Focus on the balls, not the pain**.

RHYTHMIC MOVES

As you bang one ball on to a hard surface, or bang two balls together, focus on the rhythm of the beats. Visualise the percussion musicians in a symphony orchestra playing the triangles or xylophone softly or bashing the kettle drums or cymbals loudly, as you bang the stress balls to activate different tempos.

Add another step: Include a 'blow breath', a 'huh' or an 'Aahh' sound in time with the bang. Practise making the breaths short, then making them long, and alter the rhythm of the banging in relation to the breath and sounds. **Focus on the balls, not the pain**.

SEE IT IN YOUR MIND

Bang your balls on a chair, bath edge, shower wall or table. Close your eyes and visualise the point of contact where your ball is hitting or rubbing. **Focus on the balls, not the pain**.

SEEING RED

Look at the red colour on the balls or imagine that red colour in your mind if you have your eyes closed. Chant, 'Red, red, red, red,' over and over again as you bang the balls together throughout your contraction.
Add another step: Bang the balls and say out loud, 'Bang, bang, bang,' in time with the rhythm and the bang. Try different mantras like, 'Pain out, pain out, pain out,' or anything that feels right. **Focus on the balls, not the pain**.
Note: You may choose any of the colours on the ball but chant that colour out loud.

A CLIMBING BANG

Pin a picture of a familiar image on to the wall (in my class I use the Sydney Harbour Bridge or the Opera House, as they are sights well known by us Sydneysiders) and bang your ball against the image, as though you are working your way up and over the top. If it is a bridge, move from one pylon, up to the top for the first half of your contractions (get your partner to time it so you reach the top halfway through your contraction) and then bang your way down the other side so you finish at the bottom just as your contraction ends. **Focus on the balls, not the pain**.
Note: You can also use Ayers Rock (Uluru) to do this – just use any image that works for you.

COUNTDOWN

Bang each ball separately and count, 'One two, one two, one two,' as you do. Do this first in your head, then out loud.
Add another step: Try different combinations of numbers, one to 10, or 'One, one, one', for instance. **Focus on the balls, not the pain**.

BREATHE AND SQUEEZE

On your breath *in*, squeeze; on your breath *out*, release. Keep it rhythmic and concentrate on your breath and hands as you do this.

Add another step: Practise saying, 'Release' or 'Relax,' as you breathe out and release your grip. **Focus on the balls, not the pain**.

TUNE IN

Play up-beat music and tap, bang or rub the balls in time to the tune.

Add another step: Step in tune with the music and the movement of the balls. You could also incorporate blowing, breathing and 'Aahhing' in time with your beat.

Add another step: Pin up a picture of kettle drums to the wall or floor (depending on your position) and visualise you are the drummer in the band. **Focus on the balls, not the pain**.

Cautions

- Avoid rigorous use of stress balls if you have an existing injury to your neck, shoulders, elbows, arms, wrists or hands.
- Change pain mastery technique if your arms or hands become fatigued.
- If you drop the balls, ask your partner to retrieve them. Do not reach down suddenly to do this as you'll break your concentration and could cause an injury to yourself.
- Be careful to protect the surfaces that you bang against.
- Be guided by your midwife who may have some extra suggestions.
- No matter how many times I tell the women in my classes not to tire themselves by being too active too early, I continually hear back from midwives that many women who might have sailed through labour wore out with early fatigue. Labour is unpredictable, especially the duration. Please try to use gentle, calm actions at first and slowly introduce more active ones as you need them.

Partner's role

- Check the balls are packed before you leave for the hospital.

- While she's banging the balls say, 'Focus on the bang' or 'Listen to the bang', or count in time with her banging.

- Say, 'Focus on the colours,' if that is her technique, or 'Red, red, red,' or 'Blue, blue, blue' if she is focusing on one colour.

- Give her all the reassurance you can and remind her to match the bang to the level of pain.

- Don't be shy yourself; get involved. If it blocks her pain, who cares? Bang for her and ask her to focus on your bang. Ask her to watch you, count for you and listen to the sound.

- Remind her to keep her elbows close to her body to minimise arm fatigue while she is banging. Perhaps support her hands so she doesn't tire, and bang with her.

- Put her balls down when she needs a rest from them; make sure she doesn't tire from them too soon.

- If she drops a ball, pick it up – don't let her do it.

- Get her to add extra techniques when necessary to vary the skill or if it is not working.

- If she has an IV drip in her arm, and holding the ball is uncomfortable, ask your midwife to tape the ball to her hand, so that she doesn't have to clasp it.

A story to encourage you

In my 30 years of practice I have heard many reports about the various ways women use their hands to deal with labour pain. Some of these are fist punching as though wearing a baseball mitt, a one-armed swimming/scooping action, finger flicking, squeezing bubble wrap, scratching and rubbing fabric or textured surfaces. One of my class members, Karen, rang and told me with amusement, yet awe, that after she had exhausted her use of stress balls when she was around 8 centimetres dilated, she grabbed a plastic bag that surrounded a hot pack and started scrunching it with both hands. As she began demolishing the bag her insightful midwife brought her more bags to scrunch. By the end of the labour the floor was littered with plastic bags! Everyone laughed, of course, but the amazing thing was that this was the tool she used to block the contraction pain and it took her to 10 centimetres drug free.

And now I will hand over to Sarah to tell you about her 'stress ball' class; it always makes me laugh when I read it. I love how she was initially a little resistant to what she called 'plums'!

Remember

- It does not cause pain to squeeze or bang two balls.
- The hands are typically used for expression, so *'Go for it!'*
- Banging produces endorphins.
- You can easily focus on it, especially if the ball is coloured. If you are concentrating on the balls, you can't focus on the pain.
- You can make it deliberate so that it becomes a conscious, contemporary activity. Decide to do it. Make it one of your skills.
- You can start banging instantly as the contraction demands or even a few seconds before the contraction begins.
- Banging is also good for eliminating anger and frustration, panic, fear, stress – think 'kettle drums' for extra motivation.

Sarah's story

I clearly remember Juju showing us in this class what we would look like if we froze with the pain during labour. She did this so we would have a good strong image of what huge surges of adrenalin can do to us if we panic and freeze. She tightened up, clenched her hands, wrapped them around her body and cried out, 'Ouch. Oooh. I am in pain. I can't handle it. I can't cope. Help me. It hurts.' It reminded me of being a child, when, if I hurt myself, I would immediately give up and look for my mum to help me. I needed her to fix it!

I could see that is exactly what could happen in labour. The pain starts and you tighten up, freeze, and hold on to that pain. And desperately look for help. As explained throughout this book the physiology of labour grants us huge surges of adrenalin, energy that needs to go somewhere. If this energy can't go anywhere it builds and builds and you can very easily lose control. There is a solution. By using the parts of your body that are not in pain you can deplete the adrenalin, take the focus off the labour pain, begin to master it and stay in control, and on top of this help your labour progress.

In previous chapters you have read how you can use your legs and feet, and even your eyes, to work off that fear, that adrenalin, to distract from the pain. It does seem a little impossible that by simply moving you can dull labour pain (and possibly even block it) as well as help the labour progress. But it is possible. By using those parts of your body that are pain free you are able to help yourself through your labour. The aim of this class was to again show us how to take an active approach to labour by using another part of our body that is free of pain during labour – our hands.

A huge plastic bag was opened by Juju and its contents were strewn across the floor. Little coloured balls. 'Okay,' I am thinking, 'what on earth are these for?' I had seen how we can use big movements and big vocalisation in labour but how can little balls, the size of plums, help me in what I imagined was the most painful experience I was ever going to face? We were each asked to take two balls and stand in rows in the classroom. Juju asked us to stomp our feet again, as we did in the movement class, but this time to add another step: bang the stress balls together. Some women banged their stress balls in a very fast rhythm, some in time with their feet stomping. But I was wondering, what can this actually do?

Just as in the movement class with our arms, Juju set out to create pain in one part of our bodies in order to make us simulate a pain we had to distract from. This time we used our legs as the 'guinea pigs'. Juju got us to squat down. Low. And lower. Of course, she would see if we cheated by straightening our legs a bit and tell us, mercilessly, to 'Get lower. Now lower. Stay there.' One minute. One and a half minutes. Two minutes. The length that contractions can be. It was excruciating. Don't forget most of us also had at least three kilograms of baby in our bellies as we did this!

You know when you are doing something that is painful and you actually start to feel sick? Well, the pain in my legs was big and seemed to be consuming my whole body. I couldn't think of anything else and I felt nauseous. Then Juju asked us to bang the stress balls together and, 'Concentrate on the sound. Hear them banging together. Look at the colours. Chant, "Green, green, green" or "Red, red, red." Whatever you are thinking concentrate wholly on it.' The pain seemed to melt away. My mind was so consumed by the movement of the balls, by the action of my arms, that I didn't even notice the leg pain. I knew it was still there but I had distracted myself and blocked the pain. I had also worked off that surge of adrenalin that was making me feel sick.

LEANNE *Before going into labour, I thought I would use a lot more movement to cope with the contractions. However, when the time came I preferred to sit down with my eyes closed and focus on the sound of my breathing and the 'thud, thud, thud' sound of the stress balls banging together. Just when I thought the pain could not get any worse, it did, so I just matched the pain by increasing the pace and the intensity of the 'thud, thud, thud'. It worked amazingly.*

Juju explained to us that by concentrating on those balls, by focusing on the sound of the balls, and/or the colours of the balls – such as banging the red sides together, the green sides together – we are taking our focus off the pain and on to something else entirely. We were using distraction as a way to master the pain and action to use up some of our surging energy. I remember when Juju told us to stop the stress balls activity but to stay in that squatting position without any distraction, the groaning around the room started again! We did this exercise a few times and it really instilled in me how powerful these techniques are. It seemed too simple to block something that is awful, like pain, with stress balls but it really did work.

Juju often asks those mums who are there for their second or third labours what techniques they used during their previous labours. In this class about four mums told their story of how stress balls helped them enormously in their labours. Now these are normal women – teachers, lawyers, event managers, full-time mums, etc. Each story was different but every one of them talked about how and when they used stress balls and how they really did help. Some women used them for hours. One woman used her stress balls in the car on the way to the hospital, banging them against the window while her husband counted in time with her banging to help keep her focused. Another woman used them while walking around the labour room, banging them in time with her feet stomping on the cold floor. For each woman these little balls blocked their labour pain and not one of them thought them silly or embarrassing. They understood the power of using their hands, a part of their body free from pain, to work through their surging labour pain. The stories were both amazing and convincing.

FIONA *As the contractions became stronger, I found that the breathing I was doing was no longer enough to control the pain and I started to count 'One, two; one, two' quietly to myself. The swaying I had been doing turned into a stamping of my feet, and I felt the urge to bash my fists together. My husband pulled the stress balls out of the bag. I found these were great as I was able to listen to the smacking sound as I hit them together in front of my face. I continued also to use visualisation, picturing the words 'one' and 'two' in my head as I was saying them, depending if I was placing the emphasis on the 'one' or the 'two'.*

Even so, I didn't think I would use these little balls when I went into labour – I simply couldn't see me banging them together. Still, on Juju's insistence I did pack the stress balls into my labour bag even though I had no intention of using them. I didn't even tell Juju how I felt about them – until now that is! I was already self-conscious about what other people would think when I was in the labour room doing all these techniques that Juju was teaching me and I thought I would look really silly banging these little coloured balls together. And I wasn't completely convinced that they could make a real difference when I was experiencing the big pain of labour.

Well I was wrong. Once I had progressed well into my labour, at about 7 centimetres, my waters had broken and the pain was increasing rapidly. I had managed the pain up until then using movement, by rocking back and forth on the fit ball, and using vocalisation. Now I needed something more as I was beginning to focus on the pain again. I had no idea how long I would be in labour and, unfortunately, my labour was slowing down and making me feel pessimistic about it. I started imagining how much bigger the pain could get and I was getting nervous.

I tried the bath but, sadly, the heat and the feel of the water instantly made me queasy. I was so disappointed as this was one tool I had heard so much about from other women – how fantastic water births feel. For me, though, nothing could have felt worse. I started to get worried – I was running out of ammunition. What more could I do? I felt exhausted and upset – a truly terrible combination of feelings when you are battling big pain. Thankfully, my husband was there to support me morally and physi-cally – he helped me enormously.

I returned to the fit ball, rocking and using vocalisation, but because my husband could see the techniques I had been using up until now were no longer cutting it he remembered the stress balls. I positioned the fit ball so I could lean over the delivery bed and, with my elbows on the bed, started banging those balls together. At first I was worried what someone would think if they walked into the room but the pain was starting to overwhelm me and I needed action, and fast. I bashed the balls together quickly and found the rapid movement and beat kept my vocalisation and my rocking all in sync. I had managed to find a rhythm that worked for me using three birth skills: movement, vocalisation and stress balls. I kept using them together for about 30 minutes, until my doctor came in to check on me again.

CATHY *During my four-hour labour I paced the floor, bashing the stress balls and singing 'Jingle bells', all in rhythm. It was important for me to focus only on the red segments of the balls. My husband was wonderful; he also banged the stress balls and sang as well in order to keep me focused. His mouth was right over my ear for extra concentration. The staff found it a little amusing that I would not let go of my stress balls for the pushing phase – actually I bit into one as I pushed! My wonderful stress balls are now, after two labours, a little the worse for wear.*

What is so important about the birth skills techniques in labour is that you can go into that room armed with all your weapons but you will only know at that moment what works for you. I was sure I wouldn't use the stress balls at all but they really worked when I needed them. An important message here is how those parts of your body that aren't in pain can be put into action to help distract you from intense labour pain. Although I didn't use the stress balls again, my hand actions continued to be fundamental tools for me to manage pain, particularly in transition – the hardest part of labour!

Physiologically, transition is between 7 and 10 centimetres. The contractions roll one on top of the other. They may be extremely difficult to deal with. Most women, especially in a first labour that may go beyond eight to 10 hours, will be very tired by this stage. Their thoughts may turn to, 'I want this over with.' As well, some women experience nausea, chills, shaking, fever, sweating, double-barrelled overwhelming contractions, backache, chaos and a premature pushing urge. Don't freak out as you read this. No one gets all of these symptoms at once. For every woman who has ever birthed there is a different set of circumstances. As Juju says, you need to focus on remembering that you are nearly there. For most women transition speeds things along; you don't have to try too hard to control this phase – you may not be able to anyway. This is the 'let go and get gutsy' time. Soon you will be pushing.

For me, though, my labour stalled completely at nine and a half centimetres and I had no sensation to push as my baby had moved down on to the cervix at an angle. My hands and the sensation of touch became paramount for me. At this point my contractions were rolling all on top of each other. Most women would be pushing at this stage, which can be somewhat of a relief. But I didn't have that sensation, only severe contractions with no break in between. There seemed to be no end in sight. I was exhausted, scared, and I began to freeze. It was startling how I suddenly felt a complete surge of overpowering pain and energy wash over me as the pain seemed to take over. It was awful. For the first time, after all these hours, I felt like I was losing control. I wanted to cry!

I desperately needed something to focus on. I was lying on my side on the bed. I was still using vocalisation and my husband was right there supporting me, coaching me through the contractions: 'Come on, you can do it, louder, louder, match the pain!' I grabbed on to him and pulled him closer. I started scrunching up his jumper in my hands – an Australian rugby league jumper, of all things! (Forever memories of my labour will be filled with the image of that green and gold jumper.) It was weird, a simple thing like feeling my husband's clothes, softly and gently feeling the texture of a tiny piece of fabric between my fingers, was a powerful sensation that I could focus upon entirely. It helped me through the next 45 minutes of the most forceful, overpowering pain I have ever felt. Perhaps it was the tiny movements of my hands that counteracted the immensity of the pain. It was unbelievable.

ANGELA *I paced the floor and started punching my right fist into my left hand. The rhythmic 'Aahh' sound helped more as the pain intensified. I used only these techniques until I began to feel the pushing urge about five hours later.*

It seems funny how I questioned those plum-like balls when my main distraction technique became a tiny piece of football jumper fabric! As you will read from some of the other women in my class their hands were fundamental in helping them through their labours. This technique makes sense to me now, especially when I think about other times when I've been in pain or frightened – my hands would clench up and, in turn, tighten my whole body. To relax your hands when you have more than enough to think about is next to impossible. By using them actively, through squeezing, banging and clenching these little balls, you allow your hands to be free of tension and you also help work off adrenalin and block your pain. All I can say is give it a go. Even if you just try squeezing them a little bit at first and it works, then try tapping them together. If you find that works, then try banging. It might just amaze you how this skill can really work.

MICHELLE *In early labour, at 3 a.m., I took a shower hoping that the sensations in my low abdomen increased. My husband woke up as he heard me splashing around in the bathroom. The pain had built considerably and he suggested the stress balls. He handed me one to tap lightly on the wall of the shower recess and then suggested I banged two together. This was good. It took my mind off the pain. You could say the whole labour was about my stress balls. Stress balls in the car, stress balls during the initial monitoring, stress balls in the bath, stress balls against the window sill, banging them against each other, and even clinging to them tightly as I was pushing in the second stage. They were fantastic. My advice to everyone going into labour would be:* Do not go without your stress balls.

WENDY *On arrival at the hospital I was fully effaced and 2 to 3 centimetres dilated. The contractions were becoming more painful but I was able to get through them by banging my stress balls together and focusing on the rhythm of the bang. This took me to 6 centimetres but then I hit a brick wall. The pain was much worse and I was having trouble coping. I remembered the message from our classes, 'Think laterally, move sideways.' I grabbed a large amethyst I had brought with me (to use as a visual focal point) and pushed the sharp points of the rock into each hand alternately, as hard as I could, during each contraction. I focused on this for the last two hours of first stage – on just the squeezing of the rocks and concentrating on the points pressuring my hands. Amazing!*

ALISON *Luckily our hospital supplied some stress balls as we had forgotten our own. I used only one ball in my right hand and banged it on the floor mattress. I was in the all-fours position. As labour progressed and the pain increased, the real moaning and groaning began in time to the banging of the ball. I decided it was a competition between me and the floor mattress to see which one of us would come out of it the best! It was my intention (in my mind) to pulverise the foam in the mattress with my little coloured ball. I was so focused. As the pain increased even more I had to get the big guns out. I increased to the max the 'Aahh' sound and focused on this now (while still banging) and an hour later, with the help of a little gas, arrived at 10 centimetres.*

SANDRA *The first snapshot my husband had of his wife in labour when he arrived, panting, at the hospital was me in my smiley T-shirt in the hallway of the delivery suite, bashing stress balls together, while 'Aahhing', pelvic rocking and fixing my attention on a point on the wall. I was getting through each contraction and matching my activities to the pain. This continued (we later added some counting and visualisation as extra skills) until I was around 7 centimetres. My midwife suggested a change of scenery so I moved to the shower. My husband held the hand spray on my belly while the fixed shower head was aimed at my low back. I was 'Aahhing' and bashing one stress ball against the tiles. The other stress ball I held in my other hand, and I bashed this along the handrail in a 'One, two, three; one, two, three' sort of waltz rhythm. These small changes really helped with the tedium of doing the same thing hour after hour, even though the pain relief from the balls was amazing. In between each contraction I completely relaxed on a plastic chair in the shower and just let the water run over my face and hair. We both came to realise the importance of matching the pain. We lost all inhibitions. Those endorphins really do kick in and the sense of calm in the middle of such chaos is remarkable. My husband wants to frame the stress balls!*

DANIELLE *After I had my waters broken at 4 centimetres, things really got started. I started panicking, thinking I would not be able to manage, but my husband came through. He got me on the fit ball, started massaging my lower back and counting over and over. A short time later, when I was having trouble coping, my husband reached for the stress balls. At first I didn't want them, I guess I was a little embarrassed in front of the midwives, but he insisted, so I took them. These were my saviour! I closed my eyes and concentrated on the sound of the counting, hitting the balls together as hard as I could. I continued like this for about two hours before moving to the shower, taking my fit ball and my stress balls with me. I sat on the big fit ball, legs wide apart, warm water cascading front and back, holding the handrail with one hand, and hitting a tile with the stress ball with the other. My husband was an absolute saint and continued to count from one to eight for four and a half hours until I reached second stage.*

HELEN *At home, I coped by standing in front of a fan, bashing my stress balls together and breathing slowly. In the car, I coped by using one stress ball and banging it against any hard surface I could find – the dashboard, the roof of the car, the seat. At the hospital I continued hitting one stress ball against the wall – inhibitions had long gone and my voice kicked in. I focused on the sound of my voice and the ball hitting the wall. Lying down to have my waters broken was difficult as I couldn't find a good, hard surface to bang with my stress ball. My husband was fantastic as we vocalised the 'Aahh' sound together.*

CHLOE *I'd say my stress balls saved my life. I had planned on using two, but my husband could only find one, so I improvised and tossed the ball from hand to hand, squeezing each time. This was enough (plus the 'Aahh' sound during each contraction) to get me through the pain.*

KERRYN *During the 60-second contractions I was shaking my fists rhythmically. When the contractions were coming every five minutes they were extremely painful, so I found the hard bashing together of my two stress balls to be the best distraction for me – this made me use my energy to get rid of the adrenalin. For the last two to three hours I used the 'Open' and 'Down' mantras, made the rhythmic 'Aahh' sound as loud as I could, and kept thinking I need to deplete the build-up of adrenalin to assist the release of my endorphins. At 9 centimetres I had a little bit of gas, which took the edge off the pain a little.*

ROBYN *During the stress ball practice in class I thought, 'I will never use these in labour.' I guess I thought I would be immersed in a warm bath, breathing quietly, listening to music and visualising the beautiful roses in Mum's garden. At the last minute I borrowed some balls from a friend, thank goodness. During* my 22^1/$_2$-hour labour the stress balls were the main pain-management tool I used. When the contractions were three minutes apart I needed something extra so I picked up the stress balls and started banging them to the rhythm of the music. At the same time, I was standing with my legs apart and swaying my hips sideways. The great thing about the stress balls was that I was able to match the pain level. I started quite gently then, as the pain increased, I added other elements to concentrate on, such as one of the colours. It was important for me to match up the colour with its complementary colour. I liked the visual contrast this made. Then I used vocalisation, saying out loud, 'Bang, bang, bang,' as I hit the balls. All the time I was adding to the strength with which I was hitting the balls. My husband also said, 'Bang, bang, and bang,' in time with me – it really helped to listen to his voice. For variety, he also clapped his hands loudly in time with my ball banging, which I really liked. In the end I was really giving these balls a hard time. I felt totally in control of the situation and not a helpless patient.

ANNIE *I went into labour with two things: a very open mind and my stress balls. I knew I would be the 'quiet type', and I was. I used the stress balls, quiet breathing, being totally focused, and moved through a wide range of positions. I did not want my husband near me during a contraction – too distracting – but in between I wanted him to draw circles on my back, help me relax and then prepare me for the next one. We used the stress balls as the signal; when he saw me squeezing them he knew to get away, quick smart. It worked brilliantly – a signal for him and a strategy for me.*

HAYLEY *I had packed two sets of stress balls – hard ones for banging and soft ones for squeezing in the bath. I started with the squeezing ones in the car and my husband counted with me, one to 75. I remember thinking I didn't care about the numbers but my husband realised it was better for me if he counted in time to my stress ball tapping, not in time with a clock ticking away the seconds. Once we got into a rhythm, I knew that when he reached 30 to 40 the pain would start to subside. On arrival and when we got into our birthing room I just kept pacing and tapping and counting. My midwife acknowledged how well I was doing and gently suggested I slow down a little so I did not tire myself out. Good advice as I was only 3 centimetres dilated. I modified my activity for as long as I could by focusing more on a deep slow releasing outward breath.*

JOEDY *When my husband arrived home to help me, I was already using the stress balls, smacking the yellow colours together, and making the 'Aahh' sound during contractions. When the contractions were eight minutes apart, the midwife told us to come in. The contractions were quite difficult to deal with in the car, and going around corners was impossible. I could not have managed without my stress balls. On admission, I was dilated to 3 centimetres. I continued smacking the yellow colours but eventually this was not enough to match the mounting pain. I went into the bath, started vocalising louder and hit just one ball against the tub, focusing on the 'thud, thud, thud' sound. As well as focusing on the sound I concentrated on the tiles, looking at the patterns and sometimes concentrating on the grout lines. I also counted the tiles during some contractions. All of this was right for me.*

Remember: **Focus on the balls, not the pain**.

A final thought ...

Before you go into labour, read and re-read these reports describing all the different ways women have used stress balls to block labour pain. Keep an open mind. Refer to the physiology section. If something makes sense, you will do it. At least try it. And make sure your partner knows to remind you to use them on the day in case you forget about them. Remember, Sarah forgot and her husband reminded her to start using them – and she was very thankful he did.

Whether you scrunch plastic, bang stress balls, clap your hands together or find unique ways of using your hands to help with the pain and the stress, the important things to remember are to:

- focus on the activity
- keep it rhythmic
- ask your partner to help you
- add other techniques as you need to
- *match* the pain.

We have now covered the main physical techniques that you are going to use in the first stage of labour to help you cope. Now, we need to address what you are going to *think* about. And *talk* about. And *mumble* about. And *listen* to your partner repeating to you. The reason we do this? Well, if you don't do something with your thoughts guess what they say? That's right, they say, 'No,' 'Ouch,' 'Too painful.' You are going to learn how to turn those negative thoughts around with keywords, including mantras and counting.

SKILL # 5

Keywords

So far you have learned what you can do with your feet, your breath, your voice, your eyes and your hands. In the next section you will learn what skills you can do during the second stage of labour – the pushing and crowning stage of the baby being born. Before that, though, it will be valuable to explore the sorts of messages you will have in your head during the first stage of labour, while you are having a contraction. I mean, let's face it, pain does not usually make people whistle a happy tune! In fact, the dialogue inside your mind that pain creates is usually more on the unhappy side – the 'ouch' side. But maybe there is a way you can change that *and* help your labour at the same time.

To do this you are going to recruit your incredible intellect while your body is working hard at doing something. Yes, you can have a dialogue with yourself while you are having a contraction. It doesn't have to be an unrealistically positive conversation, of the 'think only positive thoughts' kind – that usually doesn't work and only adds too much pressure – but it does have to be simple and precise, which makes it very easy to do. It's important that both you and your partner understand this.

First, a little bit of history

Ancient woman way back in time used only her instinct to give birth because her intellect, as we know it today, had not yet developed. When antenatal classes were first introduced over 50 years ago, we were taught a set of cognitive breathing exercises to help us with the pain. Then the trend turned back towards using instinct with the concept of 'just let your body tell you what to do'. Great idea, but we were left without effective strategies if this did not happen for us naturally.

The problem is that we are intellectual as well as physical beings. In fact, during the 'just let your body tell you what to do' era the rate of our use of medication in childbirth began to soar. Of course, there were other sociological and medical factors at play here, but a lot of time and energy has been spent criticising the medical system for this sharp rise in medical assistance while little attention has been given to exploring new methods for women to manage the pain of labour. What is the use of letting your body do its thing when the very clever, busy and hard-to-shut-down intellect is running a 60-second commentary with a negative analysis? This ongoing critique during contractions diminishes your ability to master the pain. Learning to change these messages and apply new ones is where the real strength of this chapter on keywords – in the form of single words, phrases, mantras and counting – lies.

If anyone tells you when you go into labour that 'your body just tells you what to do', don't believe them. Maybe it did once, maybe it still does with a small number of women, maybe it does if you have someone with you who has birthed their own children this way and you can trust and rely on them to help you through it, but that's a lot of maybes. If everyone's body told them what to do, I can absolutely assure you Sarah and I would not be writing this book.

One of the things to recognise during your pregnancy is that you will take in masses of detailed information about childbirth, but during the birth itself you will not be helped much by all this detail. You are going to need to keep any thinking messages during this big challenge simple, repetitive, and mostly focused away from the pain. You can certainly focus on the birth process, but not on the pain as it inclines to make you freeze, creating more pain and distress. You'll need to *remember* to: **Focus on the words, not the pain.**

A little physiology ...

When something out of the ordinary happens, the thinking part of your brain is brought to attention. It comments, analyses and instantly responds as part of the preparation for what might come or needs to be done. This is just another natural part of the fight/flight reflex in which adrenalin alerts the nerve cells of the thinking, rational, analytical part of your brain, so that it too may contribute to your comfort, safety or survival if necessary. In a situation of danger or crisis the fight/flight reflex and the adrenalin rush it brings with it gives you the ability, for example, to instantly cry out for help with a very loud voice. When a healthy stress situation occurs, even though you don't need to, for example, yell out for help, the adrenalin link to the intellect is still there. Hold back your vocals and you may increase your stress, let them out and you will no doubt reduce it.

What you need to do is to think of your brain as a mental blackboard. Write on it a word that feels right for you at this moment and then focus on that word. Think about saying that word quietly or out loud. As you know, no part of the brain works in isolation: just thinking of a word or words with meaning activates a region in the decision-making part of your brain. Actually speaking the word out loud engages the part of your brain involved with movement. Some mantras, such as 'keep moving' or 'keep banging', will better assist that physical activity – body activity and vocal activity naturally go hand in hand. Silent reading (as from a cue card) activates part of the visual centre in your brain, so in this situation it might be best to combine words and activities that you can visually concentrate on if you are getting your reminders from cue cards.

The act of putting words together to form phrases and meaningful sentences is confined to the left side of the brain. The problem with this is that any time you encourage dominance of the left side of the brain you also have an intellectual evaluation and critique of pain going on and, as a result, you create the production of the very anxiety state you are trying to avoid. It's best to keep away from this if possible. Using simple words such as 'yes', 'open', 'down', 'out' or any rudimentary mantras (see the exercises from page 149 for suggestions) gives dominance of attention to the right side of the brain. The anxiety state is avoided and the awareness of what is taking place is more holistic. Aim for this if possible. You will panic less.

If a word has meaning for you in labour – for example, 'open' as in 'cervix open' – it can increase your ability to be proactive in impressing upon the cervix its ability to open, keeping your brain in tune with what your physical body is doing. No one really understands the effect of keywords on the autonomic nervous system (this is the part of the nervous system that you have no voluntary control over and it also governs the activity of the uterus), but many say that using the brain to give messages to involuntary muscles can have an influence. It is, however, well established in the literature that heart rate, blood pressure and overall stress levels can be decreased using such techniques. So, if the word or phrase has no meaning to you, it can be useful for basic distraction. The trick is to keep the word/s simple and focus on it/them to the exclusion of all else.

Any form of auditory stimulation (keywords, mantras, counting, simple sounds, etc.) can change your brain's perception of the contraction pain. The louder the words, of course, the more you will bombard your brain with auditory stimulus. This, if loud enough, will override the pain stimulus and block it. Quite simply, you will focus more on your words and feel your pain less.

Strut your stuff and talk your talk

It is important that you understand that you are not being invited to express your pain with a barrage of four-letter words, although you would not be prevented from doing this if that's what you needed. Just know that civilised words can help you stay focused and in command of the pain as well as the others. Actually, it's interesting how many women do not swear during the painful contractions. Most of us would curse if we hit our thumb with a hammer so why wouldn't we say a hellava lot worse for not just one contraction, but for every 60 seconds of pain, for hours? Perhaps it's because we are so focused on getting through it we tend to stick to other, more positive or even meaningless words. Maybe four-letter words also invoke negativity and fear in us, which would contribute to us freezing. A woman who has lost control will often swear as she is now governed by negativity and all she wants is, *'Baby out, now!'* But remember, no word or expression is right or wrong: just do what releases the pain most effectively for you. Personally, I throw more colourful language with frustration at my computer than I ever expressed in childbirth! So remember not to visit me when I have a computer problem!

Your word options

Whether you are using the contents of this chapter now, during your practice, or as a skill during labour, you have several basic choices to work with:

- thinking with meaning – that is, saying 'Cervix open' as you are thinking about the labour process deep inside your body
- thinking without meaning – for example, repeating 'Tile, tile, tile', 'Red, red, red' for distraction
- whispering – that is, saying something like 'One, two; one, two', quietly to yourself
- talking – telling yourself, 'It's only a muscle working', 'Baby moving down', etc.
- talking with increasing volume – repeating 'Pain out, pain out' louder and louder each time you say it
- singing talking – taking familiar words and singing or humming them, 'Aahh', 'Oow', 'Eeh', 'Ooh', 'Uum', 'Hum' sounds
- mentally talking or spelling – looking at simple words on cue cards then closing your eyes and focusing on them in your mind, for example, 'Calm'

- listening to partner talking or counting – having them repeat 'Relax' or 'Release' or 'Let go' or 'Ten, nine, eight ...', etc.
- talking or counting in unison with your partner – swaying or pacing and saying together something like 'Keep moving'.

Your biggest challenge in labour will be to say the words with enough volume so that you can send sufficient competing messages to the brain to override the uterine pain signals. You have to *match the pain*. You have to send overwhelming amounts of non-painful messages to the brain, otherwise it will not work effectively as a pain-blocking tool. This means volume. It means turning up the dial. It means total focus on your chosen words.

Our rational brain has an unrelenting need to have everything explained and understood. This means that if left to its own free chatter as labour progresses, the intellect may start to talk like this: 'Oh, no, not *another* one!' or 'Ooww! It *hurts*!' or 'I can't stand it!' or 'I *can't* do it!' or 'Take it away, *now*!' or 'It's everywhere! *Make* it stop!' or 'Get me *out* of this!' The problem for you with this 'No, I want out' dialogue is that you will increase your stress, you will focus on your pain, and you will no doubt lose control. If, however, you are able to release your stress *and* verbally state the way things really are at the same time, then do it. An example might be verbalising throughout your contraction, 'Pain hurts! Pain hurts! Pain hurts! Pain hurts!' As long as you are *releasing* stress and not *containing* it, it's fine. Do it. Choose your words carefully though. A rhythmic 'Owww' will probably feel more releasing than saying 'Pain hurts' with perfect diction.

NIKKI *My husband and I counted through each contraction – interrupted only by me grabbing lemon oil to smell as I leaned against the bed. This was important as I always knew when the halfway point came. When I could no longer count my husband kept counting for me and I focused on his voice. The pain always peaked at the 22-second mark and this became instrumental in getting me through. We continued this until the end of first stage labour.*

Making a shift in your dialogue can totally change your possibilities. Replace negative self-talk with keywords, mantras and counting that work for you. If you are using your keywords as a primary focus you will need to harness all your powers of concentration; you will need complete immersion in your word or project. Sometimes you will have your head 'in sync' with your body, such as using your feet and repeating the mantra: 'Keep moving, keep moving.' At other times you will be totally disconnected from the labour process itself using nondescript words like 'Tile, tile, tile' as Fleur did. Her attention was riveted on a ceramic tile in the shower recess and she used those two words to create a state of mental concentration that helped her block out the sensation of labour pain.

Try to let go and just allow the right words to come to you. You don't have to remember specific words as you would for a written exam – don't even try, it's not necessary. You just have to find your own words, create your own variations, and give yourself permission to say them. It's simply another way of behaving for 60-second blocks of time. If you want to say, 'Beetlejuice tastes good,' then say it. Don't worry what others might think. How do you think my class reacts the first time I take them through a labour rehearsal of keywords, getting them to say them out loud, then making them practise turning up the dial? Exactly as you would think! After my lesson on the physiological explanation behind it and lots of practice, they eventually say, 'Yep! Makes sense, I'll give it a try!' It's intriguing that we don't feel self-conscious when we yell out, at the drop of a hat, 'Aussi, Aussi, Aussi, Oi, Oi, Oi,' at the top of our lungs but we do feel shy when we say, 'Down, down, down,' during the births of our own babies! That's worth thinking about, isn't it?

What do I do?

Keywords are another dimension to labour pain management. Use your ability to speak as it is a very powerful resource. When your labour pain is only at the level of period pain you may choose to focus right on the pain because you are curious about it. Go for it! It is not too difficult to do at this time and you will want to connect with this fascinating part of childbirth, what's happening within your body and the process you are experiencing. But if you are concentrating on the pain and start to experience more pain and more tension and more panic, it is probably time to begin focusing on other things.

When you focus on moderate to intense pain you can easily get caught inside the fear-pain-anxiety trap that ultimately leads to a loss of control. So it is important to be able to know when the pain level of your contractions starts to take you out of your comfort zone. This is when you will need to start concentrating on something else; anything that does not include hurt or pain. This could be as simple as a spot on the wall, or the music you have playing or the sensation of your stress balls as you squeeze them or bang them together. These provide physical focuses, and you have already learnt about many of these things in the previous chapters. If you prefer to stay with the contraction, as you may be using powerful imagery at this point, change your contraction word to 'wave' or 'swell'.

It is important to remind yourself that just because you may be squeezing or banging stress balls and visualising your cervix opening, it does not mean your pain is eradicated. This is the mistake that many women make in their expectations of control in labour. You see, you still have a thinking brain which is very much a part of the 60-second duration of pain. None of these techniques will work if you are physically doing them while you are critically analysing the pain. You must try to focus away from the pain; otherwise you risk getting caught up in a negative downward distress spiral, which you will find impossible to get out of. If you feel you are drawn down into the physical pain, and you are thinking/obsessing negatively about it and its mounting intensity, try to replace that critique with simple, non-judgemental keywords in the form of numbers or mantras. They can even be phrases that include the word 'pain'; for example, 'Pain out,' 'Healthy pain,' 'Working pain,' 'Pain means action,' 'Positive pain,' 'Opening pain.' Just stay away from negative self-talk.

TANYA *Acting on ideas from the classes, even though we hadn't discussed it, my husband talked me through each contraction as if we were mountain biking up a hill. He started talking at the beginning of a contraction, taking me to halfway up the hill, getting me to the top with his words, going over the top and down the other side. He did this for the whole 60 seconds of each contraction. Even though some were longer than this and some were shorter, it didn't matter. My mind was occupied enough that I was persuaded I was halfway and could get through the contraction even if it was longer. As we continued, I kept seeing the words 'Keep moving' above me, just as we had practised in class. I also added visualisation as all this was going on – I focused on the cervix opening, and I said in my mind, 'Relax and open' and 'Move down baby.'*

A good guide for commencing distraction techniques may be when you say to yourself, 'Ooww! I hope it isn't going to get much worse than this!' And you probably *will* say this at some point. Once this sort of dialogue begins, it can easily manifest in repetitive, anxious and panicked exclamations that rob you of your power and lead to a loss of control. Keywords are designed to keep you away from the 'Ouch' word and thus the 'Ouch' response.

When the pain builds, instead of thinking/saying negative things try simple reframes. A 'reframe' is a word or group of words that gives a meaningful intelligence to the pain or the stress in order to overcome the overwhelming negative response to it. It also gives you some intellectual control. Sometimes you can use dialogue that is unrelated to labour completely – it really doesn't matter: whatever helps you is just fine. In a recent class I read out a letter I had received from Michelle, one of my class members, telling me about her fabulous birth. She managed to have her baby without any drugs or stitches but the important part for me was that she typed in bold in her final paragraph: '**I loved every minute of my labour**.' Interestingly, the mantra she used was simply, 'Blue towel, blue towel.' Incredible isn't it? The point I am trying to make is that it doesn't matter what your words are. The best things to say or have in your head are the ones that work best for you.

Finding your optimal functioning level

Think about the concept of 'intellectual control' for a moment. Because you are an intellectual being, and don't just function on instinct, does it not make sense that when trying to control your pain in labour you need every bit of control you can muster? You will be working towards finding that control in both your body and your mind. Initially, you will have to 'listen' to your pain so that you can gauge the best and most effective birth skills to use.

Mastering pain and stress in labour means that you will have to find your optimal functioning level. This means the level of command that is right for you at any one time – and this will change as the pain intensity alters. Above a certain stress level, you can easily lose control but if you try to over-control stress, holding the tension and tightness inside, you can actually create distress. This can slow down the labour, increase the pain and immobilise your endorphins. You will not find your optimal functioning level, for example, if your arms and legs are involved in a pain mastery technique but your mind is focused on the pain and chattering negatively about it.

Intellectual control will be part of your optimal functioning level. You will not be using your intellect as you do in your normal day-to-day life, but rather in the simplest way possible, with simple words and phrases, to help you stay focused on the task at hand. Keywords are fundamentally simple ways to express your pain and distract from it at the same time. They are easy to regulate, not overdoing it, nor underdoing it. And you can change the words instantly when needed.

Human beings are programmed to express stress through sound and words. It's natural. It's spontaneous. Who does not swear when they lock their keys in the car? Who does not make some exasperated comment when a fingernail is broken or a ladder appears in a new pair of tights? Or curse when you just miss the bus. Think about it: these are only small and comparatively insignificant issues of stress compared with labour.

So what are you actually going to say, and how will you say it? In labour, you will have a large repertoire to choose from. You can use your words mentally, in a whisper, out loud, listen to your partner saying them or look at cue cards. Some of you will use a variety of keywords and others will focus on the same word for hours. One delightful woman from my classes sang, 'Row, row, row your boat, gently down the stream, merrily, merrily, merrily, merrily, life is but a dream,' throughout each contraction. It worked brilliantly! Do whatever suits you and, remember, some of you will want to be as quiet as a mouse, say nothing at all and just focus on your breathing, vocalising or movements, or nothing in particular.

Keyword skills

The following are only suggestions – feel free to create your own variations, although I find that those who attend my classes tend to use the same ones over and over. Practise in the shower each morning. Practise them while you practise your leg, hand and voice work. Practise them with confidence, with certainty, with courage, with conviction, for full 60-second periods – and practise turning up that dial! Many keywords can be printed on cards (or T-shirts) so you can easily remember them.

Try to take all of the ideas below with you on the day; you never know which one will work best for you.

MANTRAS FOR STRESS BALLS

As you squeeze, bash, smash (basically, wreck) your stress balls you and your partner can say any of these over and over, in time with your movements:

- Red, red, red (or 'Blue, blue, blue' or 'Yellow, yellow, yellow' or 'Green, green, green')
- Bang, bang, bang
- One, two; one, two
- Harder
- Faster
- Squeeze–release
- Keep squeezing
- Keep banging.

Focus on the words, not the pain

KEYWORDS FOR PAIN AND STRESS

When it gets harder, and you need a little extra push, try these phrases:

- Match the pain
- Healthy pain
- It's only a muscle working
- It's opening pain
- Pain out, stress out
- Panic out
- Let it go
- Feel it go
- Let it out.

Focus on the words, not the pain.

WHAT DO YOU SEE?

If you are, say, in the shower, these four-word mantras are designed so you can pick out a single word to put the emphasis on, to make you focus on the object:

- Focus on the *tiles*
- Focus on the *water*
- Focus on the *grout*
- Focus on the *drain*
- Focus on the *tap*
- Focus on the *warmth*.

Focus on the words, not the pain.

SMELL DEEP

If you use aromatherapy oil you can get your partner (as you will be busy sniffing!) to say these words:

- Sniff/smell, deep breath
- Focus on the smell
- Lavender (or 'Grapefruit' or 'Mandarin' or 'Orange' or 'Lemon', whichever oil you are using)
- *Fresh* spearmint
- You can do it, peppermint.

Focus on the words, not the pain.

WATCHING THE BIRTH PROCESS

These phrases are great if you are visualising what's happening inside you:

- Cervix open
- Baby down
- Baby turn
- Think open/see open

- Think down/see down
- See the baby turning.

Focus on the words, not the pain.

COMING TO YOUR SENSES

These are great encouragement words for your partner to say:

- Focus on the sound
- Focus on the rhythm
- Focus on the scene
- Focus on the feel (of massage, hot towels, spa jet)
- Focus on my voice
- Listen to my words.

Focus on the words, not the pain.

MOVING WORDS

Great for your partner to say in rhythm with whatever you are doing:

- Keep moving, swaying, rocking
- Keep stepping
- Keep breathing
- You can do it
- Keep it going
- Do it with me, we are in this together.

Focus on the words, not the pain.

TENSION RELEASE

When you feel tension building up, either you and your partner can say:

- Soft
- Relax
- Release

- Let go
- Go! Work that adrenalin off.

Focus on the words, not the pain.

VOCALISATION PARTNERS

Say these words or get your partner to say them in time with your action and always on the *outward* breath:

- Breathe
- Groan
- Sigh
- Hum
- Sing
- Huh.

Focus on the words, not the pain.

EXTRAS FOR YOUR PARTNER

Whenever your partner feels you need them, he can say:

- Rest
- Good
- Great
- Focus in
- Focus out
- Listen
- Follow, do it with me.

Focus on the words, not the pain.

EXTRA IMAGES FOR BOTH OF YOU

While chanting, you can think or see these images. They'll give your words extra meaning:

- Ride the wave
- Let the wave wash in, let the wave wash out
- Breathe through the wave
- 'Aahh' through the wave
- This is a big wave
- It's nearly at the shore
- It's washing over you
- Let it wash, feel its power, now it's gone.

Focus on the words, not the pain.

SEE THE NUMBERS

As you or your partner counts, you can try to visualise the number. Any combination of numbers will work. Try these ones:

- One, two, three
- One, two, three, four
- One-two, one-two, one-two, one-two
- 1234, 1234, 1234 (really quickly)
- Ten, nine, eight, etc.
- 15 seconds, 30 seconds, 45 seconds, it's over
- It's coming in 10 seconds, now five – get ready ...

Focus on the words, not the pain.

Note: I have not suggested that your partner say things like 'Stay in the zone' or 'Stay in the flow', because if you are listening to someone saying these mantras then you are probably not in the zone or flow state. When you are in the zone, you are actually not listening to anyone at all! You are deeply inside yourself.

A story to inspire you ...

My great grandfather, Peter Kemp, was champion sculler of the world. My grandmother, Australian champion. In one of my grandparents' books, *Rowing*, some elements from the chapter on coxing jumped out at me in relation to the guidelines for the partner's role when using keywords, mantras and counting:

> *There must be rhythm and timing in his orders, so that his commands are obeyed with the minimum of fuss and bother. He must never be frightened of using his voice. The more authority and confidence he gives the better. The formulas are unimportant but should be immediately understandable, easily recognised and as concise as possible...*
> *Give the command, come forward, are you ready? Paddle!*

Can you see the similarity with the cox for the partner helping the woman with her contractions: 'Starting in five seconds ... get ready ... start moving [banging, vocalising, swaying, breathing, etc.]'? I guess a coach is a coach is a coach! Sometimes in class we use the image of our own Aussie 'Awesome Foursome' – the Olympic rowers. I ask the women to imagine these four inspirational young men pulling those oars over and over again, in the presence of enormous stress and fatigue and pain. I then ask them to imagine pulling their cervix open in their minds just as they will do in labour – with the presence of stress and fatigue and pain. Of course, we incorporate the mantras 'Pull', 'Pull open', 'Cervix open'.

Keep in mind, though, for some the partner's support role will involve few words, maybe they'll need to do more massage or whatever. For example, some women don't want their partners to talk and some don't need them to coach. There are no rules in labour. The options in this chapter simply present both of you with more choice, and an opportunity to use the intellect that you have to your advantage, rather than just sitting there mulling unhelpfully over the intensity of the pain.

And now over to Sarah. She and her husband used keywords very effectively and her husband really helped her to turn up that dial.

Sarah's story

Class by now was fun for me. I couldn't wait for Monday nights to roll around so I could learn another technique to help me on the day. I was certainly not shy any more. Once class started I jumped up and into the middle of the room with the other mums-to-be, all of us chatting and having a great time, but ready for action.

Juju began as she did every class by reiterating: 'Labour pain is healthy pain. It is only a muscle working – the uterine muscle doing its job. Healthy pain.' For this class she also stuck posters to the walls with the numbers 'One, two; one, two', and messages like 'Open and down' and 'Down and out'. Tonight we were learning about keywords: mantras and numbers said over and over again to positively influence our minds during contractions. Juju stood in front of us with her rag doll, a knitted uterus, and a model of a pelvis to illustrate the birth process. She repeatedly started with the baby high in the pelvis, rotated the baby as it turns down towards the cervix, through the cervix and out through the vagina, saying, 'See the baby moving down, pushing down, opening the cervix, pushing, pushing. Open and down. Open and down. Come on baby. Down and out. Down and out.' Then she got us to start our movement skills but this time adding in the mantras.

We visualised the baby's descent through the cervix, concentrating on the process of birth, and said out loud, 'Open and down,' 'Down and out,' over and over again. Repetition, repetition, repetition. But let me tell you, it is only because we repeated these keywords over and over during the class that they came to me so readily during my labour.

JENNI *I used pelvic rocking and belly rolling while standing and I kept telling myself, 'It's only a muscle working.' I was also telling my cervix to 'Open'.*

Repetition meant I could see this motion while in labour, even though I couldn't feel the baby moving inside me. I couldn't feel my cervix but I could understand it was being stretched by the pressure of the baby's head pushing on it, coaxing it to open to allow the baby through. By repeating these words in my mind during contractions I could see the baby; I could see my labour progressing. And I could work with it, not freeze up against it. I understood why I was feeling the pain. Gosh, I totally understood why it was so painful. I knew it was healthy pain. I was proud of my body – in awe of what an incredible job our bodies actually do!

During this lesson I thought back to how unbelievable it seemed to me when I met women who told me they had 'incredible' births. Now that I was learning Juju's techniques I began to see that in order to get through labour and stay positive and, dare I say it, enjoy my labour it was imperative I stayed in control. As I was learning, being capable of staying in control is a combination of using your body to work off the adrenalin and keeping your mind focused away from the pain. There's no escaping the fact that labour pain is real – Juju and I have not written this book to pretend that birth is all puppies and rainbows! Pain is hard. It will try to combat your thoughts no matter how positive you are. But by focusing on something, anything, other than how awful the pain is, you begin to work with the pain. The amazing thing is that if you know what to do mastering your pain is possible and so is that 'incredible' birth.

JESSICA *Up until 7 to 8 centimetres' dilation I had gone brilliantly, but I began to lose control. I tried the only thing left: my spiritual resources. I got into the shower and prayed out loud for the strength to get through each contraction – one by one. Fifteen minutes later I had a pushing urge.*

An image that I know we all have of labour is of a woman lying on a bed, legs spread wide, screaming in pain. It's enough to make you yell, 'Give me the epidural!' Early in my pregnancy, when I started to get worried about what lay ahead for me, I would think about all the women in the world – indeed, throughout history – who do not, and did not, have the option of pain relief, or perhaps even a medical team on hand. I wondered how they did it if it was so totally unbearable? Now I know my fear came from the fact that I really had no idea what was going to happen to me during those hours of giving birth. Sure, I knew my cervix was going to open to allow the birth of my baby but what really happens? Where will the pain be? How will it feel? What is the pain in relation to the birth?

All these questions of mine explain why it is so important to educate yourself about what it is you are going to experience. This way, during labour you will be able to understand each stage of the birth process, to not panic, and to stay in control. My antenatal classes and pregnancy books taught me about my body – the cervix, the baby and how it moves downwards – and the epidural, where in the body it is placed, and how it works. I was also taught about caesareans and what to expect. But even with all this information I still didn't really understand the most immediate problem – the pain! Juju's classes taught me this, and how to cope with it using the birth skills.

In the keywords class we experimented with counting during contractions. We marched on the spot and counted, 'One, two; one, two; one, two,' in time with our feet moving. Counting allowed us to focus on a sound. The 60-second contraction time, which we knew by now would certainly feel like an eternity when in pain, seemed to pass much more quickly. We had something else to focus on other than the pain. By repeating the words we created a rhythm. I now know that using numbers, the phrases 'Open and down' or 'Down and out', or any other keywords you care to choose, can be extremely valuable during contractions. It can be any combination of words or numbers; whatever you use you just need to concentrate solely on it and use it to your advantage.

During my labour I moved from deep breathing in the early phase of light pain to fully vocalised sounds that I didn't stop for the entire duration of my contractions. I would use the 'Uuhh-aahhhhhh' sound over and over and was totally focused on the sound of my voice – I could hear it in my head, and listened to the inflections of it. If I began to lose focus and quieten down my husband would encourage me. I could hear him pushing me to work with the contraction by using the sound of my voice to breathe

the pain out. He would say to me, 'It is healthy pain. The baby is moving down, get louder!' But even with this concentration on the loud sounds I was making there was still plenty of room in my head for the ouches, the 'Oh no, I don't like this', and 'Make it stop'! Plenty of room. So, when thoughts of doom and gloom crept in I would focus on my baby and repeat to myself in my head, 'Come on baby, down and out, work on moving down. Down and out. Down and out.'

ALISON *When labour started, my husband and I went for a long walk. I kept chanting softly, 'Come on baby – come on down.' Later on at the hospital I was even more aware of the need for gravity, so I started chanting, 'Baby head, go down.'*

As the number of contractions increased and increased with less and less time between them, I kept this mantra going and I was able to feel great about what was happening to my body. As the pain became more and more intense I would repeat to myself, 'Healthy pain – it's only a muscle working to bring my baby down and out. Healthy pain.' My husband had been timing my contractions with his wristwatch, from the moment the contraction started right through to the beginning of the next one. In early labour I was able to tell him when the contraction started and finished. As the pain got bigger and I could no longer talk he could see when a contraction started and finished by the look on my face and my use of the birth skill I was doing – working with the pain and then stopping quite quickly when it subsided to relax between contractions.

He had worked out how long I had before the next one started and he would prepare me for it by counting down: 'Five seconds, four seconds, three seconds,' etc. I didn't have to think about when the next one would arrive: my husband did it for me. When the countdown started I knew to begin moving a couple of seconds before the contraction was due to start. This was invaluable to me as I had found a pattern to work with throughout my labour. As the pain began to increase, past about 5 centimetres, I needed all my concentration to get through each contraction, so not think-ing about when the next one would be was great.

Most of my labour techniques were done by working with my husband, but visualising my baby's descent and coaching myself through it in my mind was one technique that I had to do alone. As you read the excerpts from the other women you will see that many husbands play an active role with keywords. But as Juju always says, do what works for you and seems right at the time. It seemed right for me, with my enormous externalisation of sound, that I focused internally on my birth images. The two seemed to balance each other. I know my husband could see when I was in deep concentration and I remember during some contractions he wouldn't say anything – he would just let me focus on what I needed to focus on at that moment and allow me to repeat those mantras in my head.

ANNA *I had 10 cards with, 'Focus, you can do it' and 'It's healthy pain,' placed all around the delivery suite. I couldn't miss them. Everywhere I looked they caught my eye and kept me focused.*

I never would have learned this in any other childbirth book. The repetition Juju uses, and the picture I had in my mind of her moving that rag doll down through the cervix, was easily recalled by me when I needed it. I had clear images in my head and therefore clear messages for my body. My mind was working with my body to focus on the task at hand, not on the pain. I now see this class as being essential to work with my labour, not against it. The keywords were so much a part of the adventure of that day. You may already have strong images to take with you into your labour from what you have read in this book so far. You may be surprised what you might recall and use as a mantra when it comes time for you to give birth.

JAN *Counting one to eight over and over and saying, 'Yellow, yellow, yellow,' were our main word tools – yellow was the colour I was banging together with my stress balls.*

KERRY *My husband encouraged me to say, 'I can do it, I can do it.' In the car on the way to the hospital we were both saying, 'Open' and 'Down' repeatedly. I also kept thinking, 'Adrenalin and endorphins, adrenalin and endorphins.' I then changed to an extra-loud 'Aahh' sound to match the pain, occasionally a very loud 'Open'. We did this until it was time to push.*

KAYLEY *My girlfriend vocalised with me and I asked my husband to count, as he felt a little unsure about making the 'Aahh' sound. He would start at the beginning of the contraction saying, '45' (don't ask me why 45!) and count down to one. This was great. As my girlfriend got louder with the 'Aahhs', so did my husband with his counting. Together we matched the pain.*

HELEN *My husband would say, 'Down and open,' and he kept telling me to visualise the cervix opening. Each time I lost control he would tell me, 'Don't let the pain control you,' and 'Be in charge of the pain,' and 'Make it work for you.' He also told me to concentrate on the sound of my voice. This voice focus actually worked and I used it each time I started to lose control.*

MARIA *I said out loud, 'Cervix open,' 'Baby down' – I could hear your [Juju's] resounding voice from the classes saying the same.*

NATASHA *I said out aloud, 'Down baby, down baby.' It felt good and kept me focused on the task at hand and stopped me getting tangled up in the pain sensation.*

WENDY *I sat on the big fit ball and chanted, 'Down, down, down,' at first using clary sage oil for progress and later bergamot oil for distraction.*

DENISE *I could picture the classes and hear Juju say, 'It's only a muscle working,' and 'Think open,' and 'Relax, release. Let go.' My husband would also say, 'What was it Juju kept saying?' and I would say to him, 'It's only a muscle working,' and 'It's moving our baby down.' It worked!*

JAN *As I dressed for the journey to the hospital I verbalised the word 'relax' in a very determined voice. Sounds paradoxical doesn't it?*

SONIA *I just closed my eyes and listened to my husband as he counted, encouraged, and told me to stay focused on his voice and not the pain.*

BROOKE *Besides the birth skills making absolute sense, the 'healthy pain' mantra took on a real meaning and a purpose.*

NARELLE *I propped my keyword cue cards up against the back of the couch so I could read them in between contractions, then closed my eyes and focused on one of the mantras on my 'mental blackboard' during the contraction.*

LYN *I used 'Healthy pain,' 'Positive pain,' 'Dilating pain,' 'Rotating pain,' 'Dropping pain' and 'Go!' as my mantras. I would see Juju in my mind, leading the classes. I could also see her red running shoes! It picked me up each time; off I'd go again, changing my whimpering into strong powerful sounds. And yes, it was empowering. Incredibly empowering. I told my husband not to tell me to relax during the really strong, painful contractions, but rather, 'Use each contraction,' 'Get into action' and 'Move!' I was sure that when I'd told him to do that during my pregnancy it had gone in one ear and out the other. But no, on the day he was a great source of encouragement and comfort. Frankly, he put on a star perform-*

ance. Surprisingly, to me anyway, he was the one telling me to, 'Yell, scream, make any noise you need to make.' Incredible!

WENDY *As I neared the peak of a contraction I would make a hand signal to my husband, who would then start rubbing my back, all the time saying how many seconds I had left of each contraction. This was really good as I always knew how close the end was.*

LEANNE *My husband ran water over my stomach during each contraction and reminded me it was 'Healthy pain.' This was really important for me as for years I had only known the sick and suffering pain of endometriosis. I also used the 'Baby down' mantra. These two things kept me positive.*

KATE *Bouncing and rocking on the big fit ball, I yelled out, 'Down, down, down,' as my husband held two hot packs, one over my low abdomen and the other over my low back.*

KYLIE *For two hours my husband said, 'Open, open, open,' each time a contraction came.*

ELVA *My contractions moved very quickly from two minutes to one minute apart. My husband tentatively started to encourage me through each one. His inexperience and awkwardness initially manifested itself in hesitancy; however, this became full-blown enthusiastic support after about 20 minutes. Hearing his voice saying, 'Okay, get ready, here it comes, breathe. Let the pain out, breathe it away. You're halfway there, keep breathing. You can get there, good, almost there. It's gone, well done,' was amazing. For me the one significant mantra was, 'Match the pain with your voice'. I had never thought, before childbirth, that this was* *what would get me through. For each contraction I just got louder and louder to match the pain. It worked really well for me and distracted me from the pain very effectively. The 'Aahh' sound focus was fantastic too. Even though my husband was using the word 'breathe' and my sound was really loud, it didn't matter. I knew exactly what he meant!*

SARAH *Once in the hospital I began bouncing on the fit ball to encourage progress. I chanted, 'Baby down, baby down.' My husband kept reminding me that the contraction was also opening my cervix. It was very exciting to be so involved in the process of the birth.*

LARA *At one stage I had to tell my husband that his one-two-three-fours were giving me the 'irrates!' so he changed instantly to five-six-seven-eight. Much better! I also used the mantra 'Oxytocin, yes', but in transition I could only focused on the 'Aahhs'.*

HEATHER *'Baby down, head on cervix' – that's all I used. Each time a contraction came my husband said, 'Go.' And I did! Didn't need any more.*

MICHELLE *I said things like, 'Come on Michelle, you can do it. Don't lose control, stay focused.'*

MELITA *I used 'Healthy pain', 'It's only a muscle working' and 'Open, down, turn'. My husband said, 'Match the pain.' I heard every word, and it took on such great meaning each time he said it.*

NICOLE *'Match the pain' was part of my focus for each contraction. I began thinking it, then whispering it, then saying it out loud, and my husband took over saying it when I had to change to 'Aahh' to match the pain more.*

JAYNE *I vocalised the word 'Okay' throughout every contraction.*

TEYA *I was leaning against the sink in the bathroom stamping my feet, staring at the word 'hot' on the tap and saying, 'Hot, hot, hot,' very loudly throughout each contraction. I also sniffed some lime oil from a tissue.*

FLEUR *I found the most comfortable position was on my knees, bent over a pile of pillows. I repeated numbers, colours and objects I could see in the room, such as 'Tap, tap', 'Tile, tile', 'Sink, sink', 'Water, water'. I also chanted out loud, 'Match the pain.'*

MELINDA *I was counting through the contraction in my head – I knew the contraction peaked at a certain number and once I'd reached that number, the pain began to fade. My contractions were consistently 60 seconds long. During one contraction, I got my strategies mixed up and shouted out, 'Eleven!' I only did that once as I totally lost my rhythm.*

HEATHER *I chanted, 'How long?', 'How long?', 'How long?' all the way through the really painful contractions. My husband, holding me, would reply with the appropriate number of seconds.*

Remember: **Focus on the words, not the pain.**

And finally ...

We have come to the end of the skills to use during the first stage of labour. You may use all of them, some of them or just one of them. You'll find you will put your own stamp on them, mould them into ways that suit you best and, contraction by contraction with your partner, apply your knowledge, skills and teamwork to take you as far as you choose.

Next, I will teach you about the second stage of labour, and explore some fantastic skills to assist with pushing out your baby. Sarah will recount the story of the second stage of her labour and teach you the techniques that helped her the most, like when her husband played a vital role in reminding her to think of the coffee plunger!

Skills for the *second stage* of labour

SKILL # 6

Pushing

First stage is now over and it is time to push out your baby. At last you can actually do something physical to help your baby out of your body. You will feel the effort of the push with the reflex pushing urge: it is both powerful and irresistible, but not the 'load' (your baby) you are pushing. Sounds bizarre doesn't it? Also you will be surprised to know that when the pushing urge overwhelms you and you are compelled to push, you will not feel the cramp-like contraction pain. Ideally, do not push before this primitive reflex has established itself, and if you have had an epidural, wait for it to wear off before you push. Your body will take over completely as the uterus really kicks into gear and, coupled with the mechanism that helps expel the baby (called the foetus ejection reflex), you will not have to do any active pushing. You won't even have to think about it.

Some women may be required to do some active pushing and, as this is a skills book, this chapter will help you with imagery and instruction in how to do this if necessary, so your attempts are not just a lot of effort going in the wrong direction. Even so, it will be important to push only during the contraction and not hold your pushes for too long as this could be physiologically harmful to the pelvic tissues or cause the baby undue stress.

Essentially, with active pushing you will be helping your reflex urge if it is weak or absent or numbed, by mimicking the work of the uterus. You will do this by internalising your breath so that the pressure created in your chest will push down on to your diaphragm and uterus and baby.

Strong imagery helps as no matter how powerful your push is, reflex or active, primarily from the uterus or assisted by the breath, you cannot feel the baby's downward movement.

The reason you can't feel her is that the area your baby is in and is being moved through has very little sensation. Think about when you place a tampon into your vagina ... you cannot actually feel its presence, can you? Even though your baby is a lot bigger than a tampon, you still lack sensation in the tissues surrounding her. This is why you need to know, really know, about what is actually happening inside your body as it is working, and you need good imagery so you can help the birthing process. Protect your neck and shoulders by not pushing and straining in the wrong areas. It is also important to understand what your doctor or midwife is asking you to do so that you may push more effectively with their help and guidance if you need it.

As with the first stage of labour there will be many variations to this stage. You may have to adapt to exhaustion, foetal distress, uterine fatigue, unrotated or undescended baby, absence of a pushing urge, fast delivery, pushing with an epidural, rectal pressure, coccyx pressure, bladder pressure, etc., but you will not be alone. Your doctor and midwife, as well as your partner, will be with you. They will be guiding you and you will be problem solving together. Your partner will now play an important liaison role between you and your maternal professionals.

When pain stops and pushing begins

The second stage of labour begins when your cervix is fully open to 10 centimetres and the baby continues her journey down through your pelvis and vagina and out into your arms. The contractions continue, usually with much less or no real feeling of pain, but rather a feeling of an enormous effort of pushing on your part. The reason for the lack of pain is due to the pushing. When you are pushing you really can't feel the pain in the same way as in the first stage. The first time I show a pushing picture in my classes all of the women look at it and cringe due to the expression on the woman's face. But the expression is not one of pain, it is one of effort. Similarly, the first time I play an audio track of a woman pushing in labour, the same thing happens. This teaching tool is not to scare them or put them off, but to help the women understand that this is the sound of pushing and effort, *not* the sound of a woman in pain.

It's difficult to gauge the value or benefit of childbirth DVDs as teaching aids for second stage education. Some couples are fascinated, some moved to tears, and some want to run out of the room. No one is complacent about it though, as it is a sight that is mesmerising. But it also raises very complex issues. For starters it involves exposure of the female sexual organs. Then it shows 'opening' and 'oozing' as the baby is born – sights not normally seen. There is also the matter of the bowel, whether or not it will release some of its contents as the baby puts pressure on to it through the vaginal wall. The DVDs in my class are 'in the face' for couples. There is no escape. This can be frightening for first-time parents as there is no visual frame of reference for such an event. Some initially find the second stage class distasteful, and many cannot relate to it at all and seem quite disconnected from that part of childbirth, while others watch with awe and wonder. All of these experiences are quite normal.

I remember the night I showed the DVD of second stage labour to Sarah and her husband. (As Sarah's husband had been overseas for the partner's class, I held a private class in their home.) There we sat, watching this incredible image of a baby being born on a very large screen. I glanced momentarily at them thinking, 'Gosh, I hope these images aren't freaking them out!' But whether or not they were fazed, when the time came they were both fantastic in the way they worked through the second stage of their labour. They knew exactly what was happening, they knew exactly what to do and they applied all the techniques, especially the coffee plunger mantra and imagery, brilliantly.

A little physiology ...

The extra pushing force, also called the pushing urge, or urge to bear down, of second stage is triggered by the pressure of the baby's head on the tissues of the vagina where the stretch receptors lie. Until your baby is low enough in the vagina to stimulate these receptors, you may have a contraction, you may have some pain (remember, if there is no pushing urge and you are not pushing, you may still be able to feel the pain), but there may be very little urge. Even if you push with all your might, without the presence of a reflex pushing urge you may not get very far. This is why I encourage you to do everything you can to facilitate as much descent of the baby as possible in the first stage of labour (positions, gravity, movement, fit ball). If your baby descends well in first stage, second stage will be shorter and pushing will be a powerful reflex.

During this time your baby moves down towards the vaginal outlet, sometimes rotating a little, and her head undergoes moulding to narrow down the surface area of the presenting part, the top or crown of her head. The skin and soft tissues of the baby's head also squash up to help narrow down the presenting part. All this activity starts to open your vaginal outlet in preparation for crowning. The muscles that are actually involved in the pushing stage are:

- the uterus – it does 90 per cent of the work
- the diaphragm – held down by the internalised breath
- the abdominals – providing support but not actually pushing.

Your pelvic floor muscles during this time do nothing, so you should just relax them. Actually, don't even think about them much, other than to know they should be relaxed. You will need to think about the pelvic floor during the crowning phase, but for now, put it out of your mind.

Your muscular diaphragm is at the top end between your chest and your abdomen, your vaginal outlet is at the lower end, and your baby is in between the two, encased in the uterine muscle. The objective in second stage is for your baby to move down through the vagina and into the outside world. Think of it this way. Let's say you have had a nine-hour first stage, which has taken you to 10 centimetres – that's nine hours the uterus has been working. Now it is time to push your baby out and that muscle may like to have a little help. You cannot call upon your partner to physically help push your baby downwards, but fortunately your body has a cleverly designed system so you can help the uterus yourself, especially if it has fatigue. This is where the breath and the diaphragm comes in.

Your diaphragm, pressed down by the internalised breath, helps your uterus to push the baby down. Both it and the uterus provide downward pushing pressure when they are in action, but not when they are at rest. The diaphragm and the uterus also provide the pressure from above that will allow the baby to slowly open the taut, tight part of the vaginal opening (the part that supports a tampon) during crowning.

Many women want to know about 'the space created' between the diaphragm and the top of the uterus as you push the baby deeper and deeper into the pelvis. Because all your internal organs are nestling against each other, there is actually not a great deal of space left as the baby moves down. This is why your position in second stage may be vital to pushing progress. As you bring your upper body closer to your lower body – the ideal position for this closeness of diaphragm, uterus and vagina would be a squatting position – this potential or even imagined space is closed in and the downward pressure is maintained. If you are in a semi-sitting position for your pushing contractions, your doctor or midwife may ask you to put your chin on to your chest as your legs come upwards towards your abdomen or you may instinctively pull your legs closer to your body during the contraction to encourage a more efficient push. This brings the diaphragm as close as possible to the top of the uterus. It also helps to open the pelvis. It is good to visualise this and know the reason behind such direction.

In my class on the second stage of labour, I wear what I call my 'skeleton T-shirt'. This is a T-shirt showing all the parts of the body from the neck down to the pelvis. It is a really great teaching aid to demonstrate exactly where the diaphragm is and the action it is capable of when pushing.

What do I do?

The power you will need for pushing will come from your thoughts, the direction of the push, the pressure from your diaphragm with a build-up of intra-thoracic pressure, the powerful work of the uterine muscle, and your breath and sound, which will be internalised. This last point is quite different from the first stage of labour, when your breath and sound are externalised. You will also be holding your breath for extended periods – up to 10 seconds – as you push. Again, this is different to first stage labour. The energy you will expend is enormous, although some babies just seem to 'slide' out without much maternal effort at all – the fetus ejection reflex working at its best.

Keep in mind, you may have the sort of second stage that needs no direction at all. Sometimes babies move down the birth canal without any need for you to push, without any need to internalise breath or sound. Sometimes babies charge out quickly in two or three contractions. Some babies will take two hours to push out. None of these variations is right or wrong; all you need to know is that the options and the reasons behind those circumstances are usually beyond your control. Some of you will be pushing with all your might, others pushing with a very gentle pressure, and others will simply breathe the baby out. Again, you will not know until the day which will suit you. But with all the planning in the world, the pushing phase is, for most women, about pushing. And the pushing is done *only* with your uterus and diaphragm, breath and sound.

In labour, your medical staff will guide you as to how many seconds you will need to push for, and how many pushes you will make during each contraction (probably three to five times). As you near crowning, you may have to push through any pain in the lower vagina. You may be hesitant about this – tell your doctor, tell your midwife: they will help and guide you. And believe it or not, it usually does not hurt more to push through that pain.

Often there is a longer time between contractions than in the late first stage, so you will have time to rest between contractions. You must do this.

Embarrassment, shock or inhibitions regarding body exposure and passing bowel or bladder contents can be a real fear during the second stage of labour. There is no effective way to tell you 'not to worry about this' because if you are going to worry about it you will (I know I did!) *But,* I do want to enlighten you to the fact that on the day, when you are pushing out your baby, you are in total survival mode – every cell in your body is geared towards birthing your baby. This is where your head is. You will not be concerned with exposure or body contents. You might be now, but you won't be then. Of that I can assure you.

Things to remember

- On the day use a mirror to see your vagina if it helps. Your doctor, midwife and partner will also be reminding you where to push. Some women will place their fingers over the vaginal outlet momentarily to feel exactly where to push into, and sometimes your midwife or doctor will place a finger at the entrance to the vagina and say, 'Can you feel where my finger is? That's exactly where I want you to push into.' Even though babies come through the vagina, many women will say, 'As soon as the [midwife/doctor] told me to push as though I was doing a big poo, I knew exactly what to do!'

- So many women mistakenly put all the effort of pushing into their necks (because they can feel them), into the back of their eyes (because they can feel their faces), and sideways into their shoulders (because they have sensation there). When you are pushing into these other places you are not helping your uterus move your baby down. The whole point of having a pushing urge is to direct you to push down into the place that you have no feeling.

• The point above is also important if you have had an epidural. You will be pushing down using the knowledge of what to do, as well as the knowledge of what not to do, and bringing in imagery, and the mirror, to help you see what you cannot feel.

Pushing skills

Try these exercises once or twice to get the hang of pushing, but do not spend extensive periods of time practising pushing during your pregnancy. This can cause overstretching of your pelvic ligaments. These ligaments play a vital lifelong role in supporting not just the uterus, but all of your internal organs. They are not designed for repetitive, prolonged and non-productive downwards pressure. Once ligaments are overstretched, it is very difficult to ensure a return to normal function.

THE COFFEE PLUNGER

Step 1: Take a deep breath in. Let it out a little. Now cough. Repeat the cough, but this time 'lock in' the cough, down inside your chest as though you are trying to muffle the cough so it won't be heard. Feel the energy from your breath/cough move your diaphragm downwards on top of your uterus.

Step 2: Now use the breath and the diaphragm like a 'coffee plunger' and push both downwards towards the uterus and baby. Visualise this internal coffee plunger.

Note: This is really important imagery, particularly if you have had an epidural, so I want you to get it right.

Visualise yourself for a moment in your kitchen, pushing down firmly with your hand on a coffee plunger in a full coffee pot. Now see yourself in labour doing a similar thing using that same imagery. Your diaphragm is the circular metal disc inside the glass flask, the plunger. The pressure from your locked-in and internalised breath and sound will be the pressure, like your hands, pushing the plunger down.

Step 3: Practise doing this with your mouth closed, then open, until you fully grasp the concept physically. Then you can do it clenching and then relaxing your jaw. See which feels best for you. Hold all of this pressure for three seconds only during the practice session. In labour you may be pushing for six to 10 seconds or even longer.

Step 4: Try a cough again, but try to close your mouth at the same time. Hard isn't it? All this tells you is that sometimes when you are pushing in second stage it might be more natural to keep your mouth open with some of the pressure escaping from your mouth and throat, rather than keeping your mouth fully closed. Just make sure that you push in and down and lock in the push deep inside your chest and abdomen as you push your baby towards the vaginal outlet gently or powerfully, or sometimes a mix of the two.

THE BOTTOM END

Step 1: Place one of your hands over your vaginal outlet to check what pressure you can feel on your fingers as you cough. Then cough/push down a little more forcefully, just for a moment.

Step 2: Compare the feeling from Step 1 with what you feel when you do the opposite – blow your breath out of your body; that is, do not lock it in and do not recruit your diaphragm in the process. What did you feel on your hand the first time, and what did you feel on your hand the second time?

Note: I hope your answer goes something like this: 'The first time, I felt a downward pressure on my fingers; the second time I felt no pressure on my fingers at all.' If so, you are getting the hang of it.

Visualisation for pushing

- Breath and sound goes *in* and *down*. Don't let the breath out again, lock it in – this is vital to keep the diaphragm in a pushing position. Use your breath and sound to push the diaphragm down, like you would a coffee plunger. Take it gently.

- Visualise where you are pushing to – from the upper part (or inside) of the vagina towards the lower part (or external entrance of the vagina).
- Although you may have your breath locked in, some pushing sound will escape. It is physiologically protective to do this. It prevents a build up of too much pressure in the rest of your body. Just keep visualising 'In and down'. Think Lleyton Hewitt's tennis serve: enormous power and a long grunt.

Caution

When you do these exercises, notice how you feel in the neck, the shoulders, the throat, the diaphragm and the abdomen as you practise pushing. In fact, place one hand over all of these parts one by one and feel the tension and constriction as you push. On the day, you will need to try very carefully (your doctor or midwife will guide you) not to push unproductively into your face, neck and shoulders. Even though you can't feel the inside of the vagina, you must direct your push from the top (diaphragm) to the bottom (vagina, or even think bowel if that helps).

You may have heard some of your friends say that pushing out a baby is a little like pushing out a large grapefruit. Well, in most cases, that's probably true. So that's exactly what I bring to my second stage pushing class. A big basket full of large grapefruit! I figure that if I am going to teach this properly, then I'm not just going to skim the surface of the topic with pleasant pictures of mothers and fathers cuddling newborn babies. With the grapefruit we really have something tangible to work with. I tell the women:

Now focus on this, hold it in your hand, feel the weight of it, assess the circumference of it. Notice it has solidarity about it, but also has a little give (or moulding ability) in it. Imagine this grapefruit inside your vagina, but you are not able to feel it. Imagine having to push it down through your vagina but not having any sensory feedback that you are doing so. Imagine the pressure it may exert on the bowel or bladder.

I then put the grapefruit inside my glass and metal coffee pot and demonstrate the pushing down action of the metal disc on the grapefruit. I ask the women to place their hands on the top of their babies and exert a gentle pressure downwards.

Then I conduct a short visualisation session, asking the women to close their eyes as I suggest images to them. I alternate between the metal disc, the baby, the coffee pot, the diaphragm, human hands, fetus ejection reflex, baby's head, vaginal tissues, pushing urge, breath and sound, internalised effort ... continually replacing one picture with another, so they all become related and interrelated in the women's minds.

MELINDA *Second stage lasted 45 minutes. It was really intense and a lot of hard work. The urge to push was overwhelming and much of the pressure was in my bottom. I began pushing while standing up, leaning into a beanbag over the bed, but moved quickly to a squatting position with a squatting bar on the bed. For some reason, the first position didn't feel right. I remembered the pushing instructions from class: 'Energy, breath and thought goes in and down.' The midwife was brilliant at guiding me through this stage. Crowning came all of a sudden, and I did tear. Even though I did require stitches, I'm so glad I got to experience birth without drugs. Birth is something you can't adequately describe, it's just so powerful!*

As the women slowly come out of that visualisation session, I draw their attention again to the coffee pot. This time there is no grapefruit inside, but rather a baby doll, upside down, crown leading, and I exert gentle downward pressure on the disc, and consequently the baby. With full conscious awareness we go over the whole thing again: the internalisation of breath and sound, locking it in, coffee plunger, the direction of push (in and down), several pushes within one contraction, strong pushes, light pushes, push down low (not into the neck or eyes), variation of position, etc.

NATASHA *It was my doctor who reminded me to channel my sound in and down – I had completely forgotten to do this and was all over the place with my attempts at pushing – rather than up and out. My exhaustion was at its peak by this stage and I was beginning to doubt my stamina. However, a few light downwards pushes later – I wasn't capable of stronger ones at this point – our daughter arrived. I had a small tear needing three stitches. I felt a great sense of achievement and am amazed at the incredible physical and emotional resources we have when we really need them.*

I send the women home that night with strict instructions that that night's dinner conversation starts with their own coffee pot on the dinner table and anything solid they have at home that will fit in it – a pair of socks, small teddy bear, fruit, etc.

Note: We also demonstrate the premature rectal pushing urge that some women experience between 7 and 10 centimetres in the first stage of labour. This is the urge you pant through, **not** push with.

Sarah and her husband certainly had a chuckle as I demonstrated the coffee plunger pushing technique during their private class. At least it was a memorable technique, thoroughly understood and anchored by laughter and the glass coffee pot! We have had a laugh about it many times since, but also remarked at how effective it was. Sarah used her tools and techniques brilliantly throughout the first stage, and did not plan to have an epidural just before second stage. It was a joint decision and the right one for them on the day, but in terms of pushing and continuing her pushing technique, her obstetrician, Keith, said ... well, I'll hand over to Sarah to tell you about that.

Sarah's story

All I can say here is *coffee plunger*. Okay, I know that sounds bizarre and here is my justification: my obstetrician told me he had never seen anyone with an epidural push as well as me. Hah! Of all the things to be proud of but, really, that coffee plunger was an invaluable piece of imagery.

My husband and I were lucky enough to have a private class with Juju at our home. Juju took us through each birth skill, including her visualisation technique for the pushing and crowning stage. She stood behind me and reached around to my belly and she had, of all things, a coffee flask with a plunger in her hands. My husband and I just laughed. 'What is this for?' we wondered. Even though we were getting used to Juju's unusual props, this one was a surprise.

LIZ *After hearing my guttural sounds, the midwife said, 'Push away.' I moved on to the bed in a semi-sitting position. I imagined the coffee plunger and as a result had very efficient contractions and a quick second stage. As the baby had a dip in her heart rate my doctor gave me a small episiotomy. She was healthy and well on delivery. We were over the moon with excitement (the three stitches healed very quickly).*

Juju rested the coffee flask on my belly and pushed down on the plunger. She used the plunger to illustrate the motion of pushing in labour, explaining to push from the top, the diaphragm; not to squeeze through the middle. 'Push right down,' Juju said. 'You must lock in your breath, your sound and your diaphragm, and push down.' She repeated and repeated this to us, showing us the motion with the coffee plunger.

The pushing stage can be a bit of a mystery. The uterus and the baby do most of the pushing down work in the first stage of labour, taking you to full dilation, then the pushing urge is activated in the mother, recruiting her assistance to continue this process in the second stage. There are many analogies about how this pushing urge feels but it is odd that most of us don't really know what it is our bodies are doing during the pushing and crowning stage.

When it came near the time for me to push, my labour practically stalled. I got to 9½ centimetres in the transition stage and my husband and I were still working through each contraction. These contractions were by now one on top of the other, with no break in between. We were both exhausted. My second wonderful midwife, Louise, kept asking me if I could feel the urge to push. I couldn't. Even though I was still in control, I could feel that control slipping from me. My obstetrician and I decided I should have an epidural. I was exhausted, starting to lose it and getting anxious.

This moment was pivotal for me. I completely understood the difference between being in control and confident and losing control and panicking. It was black and white. I can now see why so many people feel they can't cope with labour from the start. And if you go into the labour experience already out of control you have nothing to start from – just one contraction and you would be saying, 'Ouch, this is painful, I don't like it, it feels wrong. What is happening to my body? Take the pain away.'

I knew I needed an epidural. If, at any time, you do opt for an epidural or caesarean you are by no means a failure. I needed my body to let go and relax in order for the baby to come to the final stage. At no time did I feel like a failure. I still had to work, I still had to push, my husband still had to support me – it was still an incredible team effort. The epidural, for me, was just another piece of the pie to help me achieve what we were there for, but it by no means meant giving up – actually I had to work harder! This is why I feel it is really worthwhile giving it a go, knowing you always have medical options to help you through when needed or preferred.

Each woman's urge to push will come at different times. This is because the stretch receptors in the vagina are low down, near the entrance, and at the onset of second stage labour not everyone's baby has descended this far down. Some women will feel the urge to push soon after the cervix has dilated to 10 centimetres, if the baby has descended deep into the pelvis in the first stage. Others won't feel the urge until much later, when the head descends and comes into contact with the stretch receptors. One thing is for sure, the uterus contracting will push the baby down so eventually you will feel the urge.

When the time came for me to push we tried to wait for the epidural to wear off but it didn't. I was completely numb. I had no physical sensation whatsoever. My husband immediately shouted, 'Coffee plunger!' I had to have a little laugh when he first said it. My obstetrician, Keith, and Louise, my midwife, stopped and looked at him too. I had forgotten all about it, caught up as I was in the emotions of my baby being about to be born. But my God, did it work. I immediately saw that coffee plunger of Juju's and I knew how my body should be pushing. I knew to bear down from the top of my abdomen, under my ribcage, with my diaphragm, and keep it moving down.

KERRYN *I had a strong urge to push and after about 45 minutes my baby was born. The urge just sort of took me with it. The midwife was fantastic and talked me through each contraction. Not only did she prepare me for the onset of each contraction but encouraged me with each push. In the end I had a small tear needing just one stitch.*

Even though I couldn't feel a thing I could visualise what my body was doing. I know that if I hadn't taken Juju's classes I would have pushed into parts of my body that had nothing to do with childbirth – like the neck and the face and the shoulders. This happens because you can't actually feel the baby moving down the birth canal, but you can feel your face and neck and shoulder muscles and you tend to push where you can feel, not where you can't. I cannot reiterate how important it was for me to have the imagery of that coffee plunger. I'm glad I did Juju's pushing class as there is no way I would have known what to do when the time came to push. I needed a clear image on which to focus. This meant that although I couldn't feel what I was doing I could mentally, as well as physically, join in the process.

KELLIE *Even though I had no feeling in my lower body (from the epidural) I was asked to push my baby out. I could not feel the pushing urge that I had read about in all the books. I was 'in the dark', so to speak. And a bit scared about how I was going to do this. My husband reminded me about the coffee plunger imagery and the 'lock it in' technique. I could not have done this if I did not know about the diaphragm and starting with my breath and sound coming 'in and down'. With no sensation whatsoever, I just mentally and visually directed my body what to do. The baby crowned without me feeling it, and she was delivered warm and wet and beautiful up on to my chest with only a minor tear needing one stitch.*

ANNA *Second stage lasted about 40 minutes and the most helpful thing was the coffee plunger image. My husband kept saying, 'Come on Anna, think coffee plunger.' It was brilliant. I pushed so hard; I could have made coffee for the whole of Brazil! After an easy crowning our beautiful son arrived. He was alert, having a good look around, and decided to breastfeed while my husband and I sobbed, overcome with the beauty of him.*

NIKKI *The pushing stage is really amazing. Once you lock it in (the breath, the sound and the diaphragm) it takes you on a ride of its own. But as soon as you let any breath escape, the ride stops and it's quite hard to push down again during that contraction as you are out of breath. Your whole awareness is about opening. I kept thinking of where I needed to push to ... right down low. With each push I got more efficient at locking it in. My midwife had asked me which position I would like to be in and I decided to stay on the bed but facing the foot of it, draped over the squatting bar, with the end of the bed dropped down. The last half hour or so is a bit of a blur now. I remembered the coffee plunger image. Our beautiful son flew out after five pushes and a small tear. The whole thing has been the most amazing and rewarding experience we have ever had.*

ALISON *The second stage and crowning took 15 minutes but it felt like an eternity. I got about two to three good long pushes per contraction. I always ended up going 'Aahh' at the end. It's impossible to keep up those sustained pushes for the whole time. I looked into the mirror to see a big black shiny head in between my legs – beautiful. The doctor and midwife urged me to touch the baby's head, and so I reached down with a shaky, uncontrollable arm and said, 'Hello.'*

KATE *By about 7.30 I could feel pressure in my back and rectum from the baby and suddenly I heard myself scream, 'She's coming!' At that point I was in the hospital but still fully dressed. The midwife yanked off my track pants and I dropped to my knees on to a mattress she had laid on the floor. I did the 'lock it in' technique, and kept thinking of the diaphragm only for about five contractions. I delivered Charlie in a kneeling position, leaning against a couch – greatly aided by gravity.*

HAYLEY *It took a couple of contractions to get the hang of how to push in the most effective way. My midwife was an excellent guide and my 'Aahh' sounds from first stage almost ceased. I remembered the coffee plunger and 'lock it in' but I couldn't believe just how hard the pushing was. The other thing that amazed me was that I could reach down and touch the top of my baby's head, which was only 2 centimetres from the vaginal outlet. I could feel he was almost there and this motivated me to keep pushing. My husband was like my coach and* now it was like I was on the homeward stretch of the marathon. He was telling me to push with everything I had as he was watching our baby's head get closer and closer to the outside world. I kept expressing my exhaustion between contractions but I was spurred on by my midwife telling me to imagine holding my baby in my arms. With the final contraction our baby was born and lifted up on to my chest. The feeling of happiness and love that I experienced at that moment was overwhelming. With no perineal tearing and with our baby and me in great physical shape, we left the hospital six hours later to go home for Christmas Eve celebrations with the family.

ELISE *I felt the pressure completely in my bottom and took the giant leap of faith of pushing into the pain to get our baby out. I didn't think I could do it; the whole thing seemed insurmountable. I felt I simply was not big enough. My doctor was fascinated (and I think a little amused) to hear me burst into the mantra, 'Coffee plunger,' and again, 'Coffee plunger'! What a helpful, clear image that was. Our daughter's head was delivered and her body slithered out soon after with my perineum intact. She is perfect. We will treasure the moments during and after the birth for as long as we live. I am so grateful for the privilege of being completely aware of the experience on a conscious level. My mother was present also and found it deeply moving and healing after the horrors of her 1960s labours. Giving birth was by far the hardest and most meaningful experience I have had and it has profoundly affected my view of life and humanity.*

JO *The second part, the pushing, was more difficult than I expected – it was really hard work. After a few contractions of trying not to push (too scared to, I think!) I remembered what to do: take a deep breath, lock it in and coffee plunger down. The imagery was excellent and it hit the nail right on the head of what I was supposed to do. I still needed coaching every so often because I was exhausted and I would start to do all the wrong things – push into my neck, shoulders, let my breath out, etc. – then I'd remember, breathe in, lock it in, push down, right down into the last part of my vagina. My doctor suggested a position change so I moved from semi-lying to kneeling upright and over the top end of the bed. That made the pushing much easier and after a couple of contractions the baby was crowning. I didn't find the crowning too difficult; I sort of 'breathed him out' with no tear.*

And finally ...

I hope you realised from the simple exercises in this chapter that in the second stage of labour most women need to internalise their breath and sound to create greater pushing pressure from the diaphragm in order to move the baby deeper into their vaginas. This is sometimes hard to do mentally as well as physically because you may have just finished the first stage of labour, in which you were externalising your breath and sound for many hours in order to help master the pain.

Remember: If you do have to actively push you need the energy and force from your breath and sound to become part of the energy that will move your baby towards the vaginal outlet. It is because the breath and sound is internalised that the diaphragm can become that extra set of internal hands to help the baby on her way.

Let me repeat, ideally, do not push until your pushing urge is irresistible. In the first stage of labour most women need to externalise their breath and sound to help manage the pain, and in the second stage they need to internalise it, to help push the baby down. So, in the first stage the breath is used to help *distract* from pain, and in the second stage the breath is used to help *push*.

When your baby's head moves right down, she will gradually open up the vaginal tissues to their maximum stretchability – this is called crowning and it is the stage we are going to talk about next. This is the time when you can reach down and say 'Hello' to your baby for the first time. Putting your softly cupped hand over your baby's head for the first time while part of her is in our universe, and part of her is still in the uterine universe, is quite a special thing!

Crowning

Your baby is nearly born, nearly in your arms, but your attention to what needs to be done right now, during the crowning, is required for just a short while longer. It may be only one to two minutes, or just a little longer. Every birth is different, so it is impossible to generalise here. Crowning, though, is usually the shortest phase of labour.

Crowning is when the full width of your baby's head starts to distend the outer vaginal tissues. Mostly there is a slow build up towards this during the pushing phase. The feeling of this is very different to the lack of vaginal feeling of the pushing you have just completed. When your baby's head crowns every tiny nerve ending in this area at the vaginal entrance is stretched, and then it is stretched some more until it is stretched to its limit. Of course this can be frightening as it is a sensation you will not have felt before giving birth. But it is perfectly normal. You have to remember that *your vaginal opening is made to open*. For nine months the hormones in your body have been preparing the area for this moment.

Preparation for crowning

At the end of the pushing class I introduce the women to the crowning class which will take place the following week. As I give them a rundown on the content of the next class, I watch the expression on their faces and think to myself, 'Oh well, looks like I will have a night off next week. Not one person in this room is going to come!' Yes, it is one of the most frightening and confronting parts of labour, and one of the most frightening and confronting classes.

No woman likes to think of that very private, special, sexual, delicate part of her body being exposed, stretched, cut, torn, in pain, etc. It's better to just block it out and miss that class! *But*, everyone in the room wants to deliver their babies over as intact a perineum as possible. Everyone wants to learn the techniques to assist this process. Everyone wants to know how to best assist their doctor or midwife deliver their baby without an episiotomy or tear. And so *everybody* turns up the following week!

There are a few things to help you prepare for this momentous event. In the weeks leading up to birth try perineal massage (see below) and repeat the mantra: *It's made to open.* Talk to your doctor or midwife about new products on the market that may help you with vaginal distension in late pregnancy. You can also practise the exercises in this chapter – those for panting and visualisation of the process. I also suggest the women in my classes carry around a picture of a beautifully intact, distending birth outlet so that every time they feel anxious about crowning they can be reassured by the wonderful visual image.

Perineal massage

- This involves a gentle massage and stretching of the vaginal outlet. Most women commence it around the seventh month of pregnancy. The aim is not to actually stretch the supportive vaginal muscles permanently, or even temporarily, but rather to desensitise you, the woman giving birth, to firm and extended pressure in that area of your body. This assists you to release your vaginal muscles in the second stage of labour when your baby's head is opening out your body. The theory is that you become familiar with the stretching sensation, and although discomfort may still be experienced on the day (although not by all women), you can relax your pelvic floor muscles, rather than tighten them, and allow your baby to emerge.

- During the massage you, or your partner, place two fingers on the back wall of your vagina and, using oils or your own vaginal lubricant, massage, stretch and generally mimic the tingling, the pressure, the burning or the pain that is sometimes felt during the crowning of the baby's head. This should increase your tolerance of the sensation by releasing, relaxing, panting, groaning and moaning with an open throat and an open sound as you experience the stinging, stretching, burning sensation. This exercise is about letting go rather than attempting to open the vaginal canal as far as it will go.

- When you do this close your eyes and visualise the area, and what is going to be happening. You can also focus on your partner's eyes as you both pant with breath or sound. It is a good way to practise working together as a team.

A little physiology ...

The feeling or sensation of crowning can be gradual or sudden and intense. The stretching and distension with the crowning phase involves the outer vaginal tissues. These outer vaginal tissues (unlike the internal ones) are packed with sensory nerve endings. The stretching of the tissues and thus the nerve endings inside this tissue may give you a feeling of stretching, burning, ripping or tearing. These are the words that women use to describe it and I am not going to protect you from them, because I want you to be prepared. Even so, I just had a phone call from one of my class members, Genevieve, and she reported that she felt none of these things as her baby was emerging. But it won't be like that for everyone.

It is important to know that during the crowning phase the feelings you experience may be just that, feelings and sensations. In other words, although you may feel as if you are splitting in two, you may still deliver your baby over an intact perineum or have just a small tear needing one or two stitches – read the labour excerpts in this chapter and you will see that it is indeed an individual thing. To put it another way, 'a sensation of splitting' does not necessarily mean the physical reality of splitting. Do not assume you are splitting just because you have a sensation of splitting. Just because your tissues may register the feeling of tearing, it does not mean you are actually tearing.

What do I do during crowning?

First you need to find the position you wish to birth in. There is no right or wrong position to adopt for this second stage. Simply find the most comfortable and most appropriate one. Most women deliver in a semi-sitting position. Some women may plan to squat but on the day find that being on all fours suits them better. A woman who wants to kneel may even find that lying on her side is better for her during the completion of the rotation of the baby's head. The topic of positions for delivery needs to be discussed with your midwife and obstetrician prior to the birth, in case there are some limitations or modifications that need to be made to your plans for whatever reason. For instance, there is no point in planning a water birth if your hospital does not have the facilities for this.

During the actual crowning, try to think of every sensation you may feel from the area as an important signal. 'A signal for what?' you may be asking. Well, it's a signal for you to relax, to let go, to be soft, to be open, to let your baby be born, to breathe or pant and to focus on the task at hand. The task at hand is all of these things. No matter what sensations you are receiving from the area, relax the birth outlet and let your baby come out.

The vaginal outlet, when stretched to its limit, becomes a little like physiological tissue paper. Treat it gently. If your midwife says, 'Push,' then give a gentle push; if you are asked not to push, then don't. If this is difficult to do, then go straight into a pant, and focus on that pant. It is very hard to push at the same time that you are panting. And if there are a lot of stretching/stinging feelings there, it will no doubt be a noisy pant, a very noisy pant. Focus on the noise you are making.

If the stinging/burning sensations are gripping you, then put your panic into the pant, *not* your perineum. *Focus on the pant and not the perineum.*

Listen to your doctor or midwife and tell them what you are feeling. Listen to their reassurance. And remember: you are nearly there. Think 'open', think 'tissue paper', ask your partner to repeat these quietly to you.

Crowning exercises

Practise the following exercises alone, initially, and then, when you are able to mentally set up good, strong images of your baby's head crowning, practise them with your partner. You will need a small mirror, some tissue paper, a sports sock and a grapefruit. If possible, I would also like you to have on hand a picture of a baby crowning, which you may have been carrying with you for quick reference at any time you are practising. No one can guarantee an intact perineum, and an episiotomy is sometimes required, but understanding the anatomy of the area as it is stretched around the baby's head and applying some helpful techniques at the time will ensure the greatest ease of delivery with the greatest care to your perineum.

PANTING

Panting involves breathing in and out with short, shallow breaths. The objective of this kind of breathing during crowning is based on the theory that if you are panting you cannot push. Try this now. Did you discover that you cannot recruit the diaphragm as a pushing muscle if your breath is moving in and out quickly and lightly? Good.

You also learned in the last chapter that to push down effectively you need to take a breath in, lock it into position, keep it internalised until that pushing bout is over, then release it, breathe in again and start all over again. It stands to reason, then, that if your baby's head is crowning and you want to avoid pushing you do the exact opposite. You keep the breath light and keep it moving in and out. Try both now and compare the two opposites.

Step 1: Refresh yourself on the pushing technique: lock in the breath and push down into the vagina for just a few seconds.

Step 2: Now focus on the panting technique: breathe with quick, light breaths for just a few seconds.

Note: On the day you can slow down the pant if a faster pace is not needed, but keep it shallow if the stinging and burning is a problem. At this point in labour most women will need to pant and breathe the baby out rather than push it out, but be guided by your doctor or midwife as you won't know what exactly is required until the day. **Focus on the pant and not the perineum**.

TISSUE PAPER IMAGERY

Step 1: Hold a piece of tissue paper (toilet paper is a little too soft) in front of you between both index fingers and thumbs. Pull it apart until it tears a little. Notice how easy it is to do this.

Step 2: Now take a new edge of the tissue paper and pant lightly as you exert as much pulling tension as you can, slowly and gradually, but without the paper tearing.

Note: If you do this over a 60-second period you will see that your piece of tissue paper has actually stretched a little. Just a little! If it tears, just start again – it usually takes a little practice. The lesson to be learned with this exercise is to appreciate the delicate nature of your vaginal outlet during crowning. When the tissues are so stretched they are thin and fragile. Too much pressure (if you push rather than pant) can cause them to tear, but gentle, gradual pressure (you panting, and the uterus pushing) may secure that extra little bit of diameter needed for your baby to be delivered with your perineum intact.

Add another step: Try this again – pull the tissue paper apart (without tearing), keeping the tension, increasing the tautness between your fingers. Then close your eyes, keep panting and listen to your partner whispering, 'Tissue paper, tissue paper.'

Note: You should realise that you can stretch something very delicate, which seems like it should tear, just a little bit more. In labour, you may need only that little bit more stretch for your baby to slip out of your body without tearing to the perineum. **Focus on the pant and not the pain**.

THE GRAPEFRUIT AND SOCK

Step 1: Place a grapefruit deep inside a sock (a large orange will also work well) and pant as you slowly press the grapefruit out to the opening of the sock. Notice how the folds of sock stretch around the fruit.

Step 2: Pant as you press out again, then relax the sock a little around the grapefruit before panting and pressing again. Notice the sock stretch so that you will see a little more of the grapefruit each time. Relax the pressure again so that the grapefruit slips back inside the sock a little.

Step 3: Repeat these two activities (the pressing and the slipping back) until the sock outlet eventually opens fully to the widest diameter of the grapefruit.

Note: It is important to understand that there is a similar 'slipping back' activity of the baby's head during crowning. What can be frustrating is if the baby's head continually slips back the same distance you have just pushed it out. Your muscles need gentle and gradual stretching in order to stretch without trauma. Be patient. Play a conscious role in assisting the crowning process. There will be progress leading up towards crowning and there will be slipping back. In most cases this physiological activity will assist the stretching process. Listen to your doctor and midwife and try to do exactly what they are asking, even though you are at the end of your tether and want it all over – and you don't care how!

Add another step: Return to your crowning grapefruit for a moment. Slip your finger under the edge of the stretched sock. Feel how thin it is, how taut it is, how delicate it is – just like tissue paper – and as you watch this, pant, and tell yourself: '*It's made to open*.' Now close your eyes and say to yourself, 'Just a little more, be gentle, just a little bit more ... a little more stretch, relax, open, yield, just a little bit more.' **Focus on the pant and not the panic**.

WATCHING YOURSELF

As you practise panting, look at your face in a hand mirror. Your face is relaxed, your lips may be relaxed or pursed (if you prefer a 'blow pant'). Look at this image of yourself over and over again. What do you look like? Remember, you are not pushing – you are panting.

Note: If all your crowning strategies fail on the day, and the perineal pain and the panic grip you, just work at reproducing the facial expression you have right now. Keep practising this over and over in the last weeks of pregnancy. Use the mirror for visual feedback. **Focus on the pant expression, not the pain.**

We have just talked about crowning as if you can *feel* it. But many of you will have had an epidural administered and will *not* be able to feel it. Your doctor and midwife will let you know what is happening, and your partner will do the same. If it is appropriate and you want to, you can use a mirror to watch the crowning and birth yourself, but don't dwell on this if you don't want to. It doesn't matter. You can still imagine the birth in your mind just as you would wish to see it. Soon your baby will be out and in your arms; then you will have plenty to see! And plenty of warm, wriggling feelings to feel. And the touch of your baby's skin on yours. You will soak up your baby's gaze as she lies on your chest and take in the expression on your partner's face, all with awe and wonder. It is such a beautiful time. So do not allow yourself to have doubts about decisions you make. You need to do what is right for you and the baby.

As second stage started for Sarah and her husband, an epidural, administered at $9^{1}/_{2}$ centimetres, had taken effect. But with the same teamwork, the two of them managed to do what needed to be done in order to bring their beautiful baby boy into the world. Their story will help you understand the experience and you will learn from them.

Sarah's story

The crowning is the point in the labour journey when you are very close to meeting your baby. This is the moment when your midwife or doctor will tell you to stop pushing and start panting. It is very important during this stage to focus on both what you are feeling and any instructions given by your midwife or doctor. The techniques required during the crowning are very different from the active management of pain during the first stage and also different to pushing. Now you have to pant, to relax, and to let it open.

During crowning it is important to pull back on any forceful breathing and just take short sharp in and out takes of breath. Your focus will move on from the coffee plunger image to ones that will assist the softening and relaxing of your vaginal outlet so that it opens for your baby to emerge. To demonstrate the crowning Juju had a grapefruit inside a sock and showed us how the head of the baby (in this case, the grapefruit) comes out of the vagina (sock) and can fall back a little. She also handed to each of us in the class a piece of tissue paper. We were asked to hold the tissue paper between our fingers and to gently pull it apart. During this tugging or pulling of the tissue paper we were instructed to close our eyes, to focus on the paper in our hands and to pant. Tissue paper was ripping all around the classroom and women were laughing. Despite the merriment, we were learning a valuable lesson.

Feeling the fineness of the tissue paper and how easily it could tear was a strong image for us to understand what happens and could happen to our bodies during birth. We could see and feel the tautness of the paper, and how delicate the balance is between pulling it apart with force or stopping and panting, allowing the paper to remain taut without tearing. Juju said, repeatedly, 'Think of tissue paper.' And then she would rip it in two. 'Ouch,' we thought (and some said out loud). We could almost physically feel it. And then she would add, 'Stretch the tautness,' pulling the paper so far that it started to stretch, but not allowing it to rip by stopping and panting. It's amazing just how much stretch you can get from tissue paper without actually tearing it!

SHARON *The urge to push continued and I tried to visualise the coffee plunger. It helped enormously and with three or four pushes, my husband could see the baby's head. The second midwife handed me a mirror and I watched in amazement as his head appeared. As the midwife told me not to push during crowning, my husband reminded me of the mantras 'Tissue paper' and 'It's made to open'. Once his head was clear and the cord removed from around his neck, my husband took over and delivered him straight on to my belly. He was warm and slippery and screaming! After the placenta was delivered, I got up, showered, feeling exhausted, but triumphant! Not a cut or tear to be seen.*

Juju did this exercise with the tissue paper over and over again during the class. So much so, that when it came to the crowning stage of my labour I could see the tissue paper and I immediately stopped and relaxed as much as I could. Juju taught us that our bodies are made to open. Because I had no sensation here as the epidural had not worn off I had to concentrate entirely on what my obstetrician and midwife were telling me to do. They would direct me about when to push and when to just pant and relax. At this stage Keith, my obstetrician, asked me if I would like a mirror to help me see the baby's head crowning. At first I didn't want to as all I could focus on was giving birth. But then I remembered the whole reason I was there: my baby was about to be born and I couldn't wait to see him. The mirror helped me to see exactly where I was in the birthing process and to help me take direction from my medical team.

Many women say they feel a burning or tingling sensation as the baby's head stretches the delicate vaginal tissue. Some even feel like they are tearing but this is not always the case. Because it just might sting or burn for you, you may need to distract yourself from the sensation by focusing on your panting, on relaxing images or on the tissue paper visualisation. Remember, you are nearly there. Any moment now you will be seeing your baby.

MELITA *I remembered Juju's coffee plunger image for second stage and just tried hard to push down and not let the energy get stuck in my neck. I took a little picture of a coffee plunger with me. I didn't actually look at it in labour, but imagining it reminded me of how to push. During the crowning contractions I felt near panic as I didn't feel I could stretch any more. I asked the doctor to guide me through every moment. He did and with some small pants and pushes my baby girl's head finally came out. I only had a small tear.*

This class also focused on us as a group talking about a part of our body that is usually so very private. Most people are uncomfortable with talking about this part of their body, and this may be why we often don't know what to do at this stage of our labours. At this point I have to write a little bit about the possibility of a bowel movement during birth. It is the something we all fear – come on, I know you do. When talking with my girlfriends before my birth we would all squirm at the suggestion and quietly think, 'Yuk, what if I make a bowel movement on the bed during birth?' Well, honestly, it is the last thing you worry about during birth. Firstly, you don't give birth on a pristine white-sheeted bed. Your delivery bed will have your blood, amniotic fluid and I don't know what else on it, and no one will notice a little bowel movement, if it happens. And secondly, at the moment of birth it is the last thing on anyone's mind – yours, your partner's, your midwife's and your doctor's. What you are thinking about is the baby, and its first breath of life. So if you were worried about this one graphic little detail put your mind at rest. It is so not important at the time. This class allowed us to laugh and have fun but also to leave feeling confident and educated and with strong visual images about birth. By attending Juju's birth skills classes I had achieved something pretty amazing. I had eradicated my fear of childbirth. I had learned so much about my body during labour as well as what my baby was doing during labour. I changed from someone dreading the big day and just wanting it to be over, to someone who was actually looking forward to giving birth. What's more I know that each and every woman in those classes with me also felt this way.

LOUISE *My midwife telling me to 'push like crazy' was like a green light to let go and do something positive rather than trying to distract from the pain. There is nothing on earth that sounds like a woman pushing out a baby! After 30 minutes, our beautiful son was born. It was so help- ful knowing the right thing to do. There is very little sensation to tell you what you are doing and having clear and simple images in your head tells you exactly what to do – and what not to do. I touched my baby's head as he was coming out (my husband told me he had dark hair) and it felt wonderful. I will never forget how good he felt. I only had two stitches from internal grazing, but my perineum was intact.*

At the end of each term Juju asks a few couples who have been through the birth process and used her birth skills to come in and talk to her present class members and their partners. We listened intently as they told us about their incredible births and adventures. These couples looked at us with excitement, not the pity I had previously experienced. I am now one of them, having given birth using the birth skills, and as you will read in 'The bigger picture' section, I do not tell a story of an horrific experience: exactly the opposite. As we said our good lucks to our fellow class members we looked at each other with excitement and pride, and great anticipation for what lay ahead of us.

DANA *Juju's classes changed my life. The birth of my first child, my beautiful three-year-old daughter, was full of interventions that left me both physically and emotionally traumatised. It was 12 months before I could sit down properly after the birth! This time after learning the birth skills, which I didn't know about* the first time around, I delivered our son, who was 3.1 kilograms, naturally and drug free. Late in transition I got into the shower as the contractions were really intense. At this point I heard a change in my voice during contractions; I could actually hear myself making a pushing, groaning sound and felt an urge to empty my bowel. The midwife told me it was okay to push now. As I got out of the shower I had one extremely intense contraction as I was leaning over the hospital mobile tray and my waters broke – unfortunately, all over my husband's jeans and shoes! I got on to the bed on my knees, facing the wall, and started pushing. My doctor had arrived and I continued bearing down as I listened to my husband's amazingly encouraging words as he held my hand. I did tear a little along my old scar, but that was nothing in the whole scheme of things.

NICOLE When I looked into the mirror I got some supernatural force from somewhere. I pushed as hard as humanly possible and then a bit more on top of that with each contraction. There was no pain at this stage. I could see the baby's head reflected back at me, and I could see her advancing towards the vaginal outlet more and more with each push. There was a small amount of retracting of her head, but this allowed my muscles to stretch gently, so it wasn't a problem. I was able to push easily like a coffee plunger and just use the muscles needed. I completely relaxed my arms and legs. My doctor knew that I wanted to avoid an episiotomy or tear, so I really worked at pushing out my baby's head even though I could feel an intense stinging sensation at the vaginal outlet. I used the mantra: 'I am not tearing, just relax' as I remembered you [Juju] told us that a sting does not mean a tear ... it just means a sting. This is what I focused on and I blocked everything else out just for a few contractions. Her shoulder emerged with the next push, then our little girl shot out like she was coming down a water slide! As soon as the head and shoulders were out, I got this huge rush of natural endorphins. I felt incredible and there was no lingering pain at all. My perineum was intact. I was on a high for days afterwards, I did not feel tired at all, and we are still celebrating the arrival of our beautiful baby girl.

JAN *The baby was coming quickly. I managed to remember 'lock it in' as I pushed. I changed immediately to panting when my midwife instructed me to, and focused only on this. I gave birth two hours after arriving at the hospital.*

KATYA *I started to feel a pushing urge and got on the floor mattress on all fours. At first I didn't feel I was getting anywhere – it was so frustrating. Suddenly, though, an even stronger pushing urge kicked in (I'm not sure if the first one was only rectal sensations rather than vaginal) and I could really feel the coffee plunger working. I really felt the burning, stinging and tearing sensation of crowning and was convinced I was ripping. Just as she was crowning, I had to stop pushing as the cord was wound tightly around the baby's neck. My midwife released it and I could push again. Two more gentle pushes and she was born. I was amazed to discover I had delivered her over an intact perineum. Not one stitch. My husband was a bit hesitant, but eventually excited, to cut our baby's cord.*

WENDY *The second stage contractions were four minutes apart, so in between them we were talking, laughing and joking. When the contraction came it was all up to me and I had to use my mind to focus on how to push. I stopped the pain noises and started the pushing noises – 'in' and 'down' and 'lock it in'. I felt I was pushing the baby out for an eternity but it was only 15 minutes. At last the head started to crown and, yes, all those burning feelings were there. The* burning turned into stinging and ripping sensations. I yelled out in panic, 'I'm crowning!' 'Yes, you are,' said the midwife. I began pushing and focusing on 'open', 'relax', 'stretch' and the mantra 'It's made to open'. What a relief when she was born and placed on my abdomen. I had only a slight graze, no stitches. For a few silent seconds we just stared at each other. I stared at her with fascination, and it seemed she was doing the same at me. Unbelievable!

ANNELIESE *We'd been told to expect a big baby and lots of stitches. At 10 centimetres, there was an explosion (my waters breaking) and a tremendous urge to push. So the pushing and panting phases began and the potential for my greatest fear – so many stitches I wouldn't be able to sit down for a month – to come true. Visualisation was the key. The tissue paper imagery from the crowning class was what I used. Visualising the tissue paper stretching without tearing was my 100 per cent focus … and the outcome was nothing short of a miracle in my books: an intact perineum and zero stitches!*

TANYA *In second stage I needed to be reminded of the coffee plunger. The pushing phase felt very different to earlier contractions and although the contractions were painful there was enormous pressure in my rectum and I could feel my perineum stretching. All the time, my husband talked me through contractions and encouraged me to keep going. While the obstetrician was instructing me to push three times during each contraction, the intensity seemed to only help me through two pushes, so I had to summon the third one from deep inside me. The groan that came out was pure animal, but I wasn't embarrassed. Our midwife said, 'You aren't tearing – keep pushing.' I think I only thought of the tissue paper image once, but that was enough! After eight hours of full-on labour I delivered our baby boy over an intact perineum. I was* fully awake and aware, absolutely exhilarated and excited. Yes, there were times we were close to the limits of what I could bear, but the techniques really helped us control the situation. My husband had always said, 'Just keep an open mind about pain relief. You may not be able to have a drug-free birth and I don't want you to be disappointed.' In the end, I was so proud of myself for having the birth experience I could have only dreamed about, without any pain relief. I felt empowered, and in a moment of endorphin-filled madness said: 'I would do that again!'

HELEN *Second stage was only 30 minutes with the head crowning after a couple of contractions. I felt great frustration hearing everyone talking about this brown-haired head, as by the time I opened my eyes to look in the mirror she had slipped back inside again. My fabulous midwife stretched my perineum a little and controlled the crowning perfectly so I had no tearing. I am so glad I had the knowledge and confidence to be able to push it to its limits.*

ANDREA *Finally I was fully dilated. I got off the bed and squatted on the floor mattress with my husband sitting behind me, supporting my arms on his knees. The contractions were incredible. No pain, just this powerful pushing activity. The opening of the vaginal outlet with crowning and the burning sensation that came with it was eased by remembering the mantra 'Open and relax'. So I managed to get him out – all 4.5 kilograms of him – with only one stitch for a small tear. It was exhilarating to finally hold him.*

FIONA *By 9.20 p.m. the doctor arrived and I started pushing properly, imagining that strong image from classes: trying to visualise the coffee plunger and locking in each push. I found this second stage of labour very difficult, particu-*

larly close to the end when I could feel the baby slipping in after each contraction. It was just so disheartening to feel all that hard work slipping back. I continued to clutch the stress balls tightly in my hands throughout this second stage, just for security. I became pretty exhausted and my legs in particular were very tired, so I moved on to my left side, holding my right leg in the air, and immediately felt more comfortable. The midwife was particularly encouraging and my husband was wonderful too. He was standing and moving from where he could talk to me and encourage me, but then actually see our baby being born. Once the head was crowning I was told that the baby had lots of dark hair and reached down to touch the head. The most bizarre sensation I felt was when I had pushed the head out and I could still feel our baby kicking and squirming inside me. One more push and the shoulders and the body were out and the doctor put the baby up on the bed where I could see her. I was able to be the one to say, 'It's a girl!' as my husband cut the cord.

And finally ...

Your baby is born.

This is what you have been working towards. It is the reason you bought this book. It is a time to celebrate. But I would be remiss if I didn't make a few observations about this time.

After your baby is born, the third stage of labour takes place. This involves the delivery of the placenta. Most of you will not be aware of this activity as the baby will be in your arms and be the focus of your attention. Occasionally this stage needs to be medically managed; if so your medical team will be there to support you and tell you what is occurring. You may need stitching up of your perineum after this stage.

You have no doubt heard that the feeling of giving birth and at last holding your baby in your arms is the most magical experience you will ever encounter. Well, it might be, and on the other hand it might not be. Sometimes your expectations may be too great, or you might be too exhausted to feel anything, especially if your labour has been long and difficult (just get that first cup of tea: it'll taste great!) Sometimes the effects of an epidural can interfere with your hormonal component of bonding and you may feel almost devoid of feeling. Conversely, you may have had a very fast, intense, overwhelming labour and may need recovery time from the shock before you are able to feel loving again. All of these possibilities are normal. Don't feel guilty. Give yourself time, you deserve it. You've just given birth and that is a huge thing.

Open as much as you can to this moment. You will never see your child quite like this ever again. Look at your partner's face. You may never see his expression quite like this again. Close your eyes and really feel this momentous occasion. Besides childbirth being an intensely physical act, there are many feelings that will flood you all at once. So much so that you may only be able to articulate simple things like, 'Hello, baby.' 'Hello, darling,' 'Oh,' 'Is everything all right?' It truly is a feeling time, not a talking time.

The cutting of the umbilical cord is a ritual in itself. This may have significance for you, or it may not. Your partner may cut the cord if he wishes. Your doctor or midwife may offer him the choice. The cutting of the cord heralds the final physiological separation between mother and child. This is why it sometimes becomes an important issue as to who has this responsibility and who values the participation.

So now you and your partner are faced with a 'Goodbye' and a 'Hello'. It is goodbye to the nine months of life with your baby in utero and it is hello to a wonderful new life that will involve the three (or more) of you as a family.

You have come to the end of the birth skills that Sarah and I want to share with you. Read them over and over again. *Remember*: repetition, repetition, repetition! It's the best way to learn.

In the next chapter I will be encouraging you not to read but to get down on that floor and start to practise, practise, practise ...

Practice *and* preparation

PRACTICE

Make sure you know your skills

You do need to make time to practise your activities for labour. You can achieve this easily by doing the exercises, thinking about them so they are in your mind while you are on your way to work or the shops, or even while you are in the shower every morning. You also need to make sure you have all your props and tools ready to take with you to the hospital, and your chosen or created CDs and cue cards at hand.

By practising the skills you will get used to them, so that any inhibitions you may have about doing them are dealt with. I have already mentioned that as well as the labour rehearsal work we do in the classroom I take my groups out into the stairway, the lift, the car park, the street and the mall – even outside a well-known coffee shop. By the time the women go into labour they have no problems with inhibitions and using their skills. A positive attitude is not enough to get you through childbirth. The best plans and techniques in the world will not work for you if you are too shy to use them on the day!

Think 'solution'

Recently I watched an interview with Yurik Sarkisian, the champion Armenian-born Australian weightlifter. Wow, what a guy. I was riveted by him as he talked about how he focused during competition. He said,

'When I am lifting, I see nothing, only the bar. If you put my whole family in front of me I would not see them. I only see the bar.' When Sarkisian is lifting his weights he is focusing on the lift, the solution, as he labours with his load.

I want you to think about this, not only as you are practising but, more importantly, while you are in labour and dealing with each contraction. As part of your practice imagine you are having a painful contraction in your forthcoming labour. The first few seconds will be about the 'problem' and the 'panic'. The next 55 seconds are about your 'solution'. Everything you do will need to be focused on moving through the contraction with the skills you are using as you labour with your pain.

Use everything you have learnt in this book as you and your partner practise together. Put everything from each chapter together now, so that the parts that you have learnt now become whole. Add passion and drama so that all that is unfamiliar becomes familiar. It has been said that every experience in life is a 'little drama', so don't hold back with your experience of mastering the pain. Practise over and over – mentally and physically.

On the day, it will not be the skills that will be your greatest challenge; it will be overcoming your natural tendency to freeze. The following 25 labour skills will help you to think totally about the solutions. *Remember*: **Action, action, action ... Rhythm, rhythm, rhythm ... Focus, focus, focus ... Solution, solution and solution!**

Pelvic floor exercise

If you are attending pregnancy exercise classes, yoga or Pilates classes, aqua fitness classes, etc., you may be doing this already as part of your routine. If not, do the following 20 to 30 times each day until birth:

- squeeze your vaginal and rectal muscles inwards and upwards for five to 10 seconds. Then relax.

You can also do a quick version, squeezing for one or two seconds, then relax.

Practice skills

All of the following 25 exercises will help you practise for the first stage of labour. Try two or three of them each day. When you get to the end of the 25 start over again, repeating two or three daily until the end of your pregnancy. Practising three exercises a day will only take about three minutes and they can be spaced out over your day if it's easier – one in the shower in the morning, one at lunchtime and one after dinner.

I have not included any second stage pushing or crowning exercises in this section, as I do not want you to be doing repetitive pushing or straining activities during pregnancy. Even though you will have tried many of the exercises throughout the previous chapters, you would have practised most of them in isolation. I now want you to start putting all the skills together so that they seem a little more realistic – position plus breath plus leg activity plus hand activity plus smell plus mental imagery, etc.

As well, it is important to practise them together to establish the sort of teamwork you will need, and also to start giving your partner feedback on his role: Does his massage need to have more pressure? Does he feel comfortable counting as you sway or stamp? What are the best trigger words between the two of you for visualisation? Check that he doesn't get dizzy when breathing or blowing with you. Does he feel embarrassed saying the 'Aahh' sound with you? There is so much to learn not only about labour, but also how the two of you will relate to one another.

I have specifically incorporated different positions for your practice, although you won't know which ones you will favour until the day as you will experiment with different positions during labour, and can refer back to each skill chapter for ideas and quick visual reference. The practice sessions here will help train you to make focusing second nature. This is vital. So many women go into labour and attempt to be active but end up focusing on the pain. They eventually freeze and move into panic and loss of control. Regular practice will help you form a reliable pattern of focusing on your chosen pain-blocking activity and *not on the pain*.

Although the exercises are quick 60-second practice sessions, don't forget to linger at the end of each exercise and rest for a moment. This is just as important as the 60 seconds of activity.

WHILE STANDING

1. Sway your hips from side to side and bang stress balls together rhythmically, like a light clap. Focus on the sway then the bang. Then rest.

2. Step on the spot while you count one to 10, over and over. Focus on your feet and counting. Now rest.

3. Rhythmically and gently bend and straighten your knees a little, and rub your low abdomen with both hands in a circular direction. As you do this, blow rhythmically, visualising that you are blowing out birthday candles on a cake with lime icing. Your partner can hold a tissue dabbed with lime aromatherapy oil – it's delicious to smell – to heighten your visualisation. Focus on your movement, then the rub, then the breath. Then rest.

4. Hold a hot pack on your belly and sway from side to side and count 'One, two; one, two' in rhythm to the sway. First count to yourself in a whisper, then out loud, then with your partner. Focus on your sway and counting. Then rest.

5. Press your back against the wall and move your body up and down the wall gently and rhythmically saying, first to yourself and then out loud, 'Down, down, baby down.' While doing this, smell a tissue dabbed with three drops of lavender oil at 1-second, 15-second, 30-second and 45-second intervals. This will move you through the 60 seconds that a contraction takes. Focus on the movement, then the mantra and then the smell. Then rest.

6. Lean against a sofa, bench, sink, etc. for support and repeat the mantra: 'Healthy pain,' while you sway rhythmically. Focus on your sway then your voice. Now rest.

7. Pace up and down your hallway/room and chant rhythmically, 'Keep

moving, keep moving.' Try counting your steps. Focus on your steps then the mantra/s. Now rest.

8. Lean against the bonnet of your car, breathing and relaxing. This is to practise for the journey to the hospital, and for any contraction you may have before you get into the car or at the car park when you arrive. Focus on yourself, and only yourself! Now rest.

9. In the shower, stamp your feet while holding a flannel dabbed with mandarin oil. Smell the scent as you breathe in rhythm to the stamp. Focus on your legs or the smell. Now rest.

10. In the shower, bang your stress balls rhythmically against the wall tiles. As you do, breathe, then say 'Aahh' or count, and stamp, rock or sway as you prefer. Focus alternately on your actions and rhythm. Now rest.

WHILE SITTING

11. On a chair, lean forwards with your elbows on your knees. Relax your hands across your lap. Breathe in normally, and then breathe out through pursed lips while you think 'feather-light breath'. On the next breath out think 'breeze', breathing out more strongly. Focus on your breath, especially the one out. Then rest.

12. Sit on a chair facing backwards with your arms resting on the back of the chair. Hold your stress balls gently in your hands then squeeze and release the balls. Breathe in for the squeeze. Breathe out for the release. Focus on the balls then your breath, especially the release of your hands and the release of your outward breath. Now rest.

13. Gently bounce on a fit ball and say a light 'Aahh' in rhythm with the bounce. If your shower is big enough, take the ball in there. First, feel the water on your back, then on your abdomen. Focus on the sound of the 'Aahh', then the movement, then the feel of the water. Now rest.

    Note: Do not do this if your baby is in a posterior position.

14. Sit in the passenger seat of your car, and breathe in rhythm as you count and tap your stress balls. Focus on your actions alternately. Now rest.

15. In the passenger seat of your car, relax and concentrate on your CD. Focus on the sound – the music or the voice if it is a visualisation script. Now rest.

KNEELING

16. Kneel and rub your low abdomen lightly with the palm of one hand. In your other hand hold a lavender-scented tissue. Blow towards a visual focal point in the room and as you do so, take in the scent of the tissue. Focus on the blow then the focal point, as well as the smell. Now rest.

17. Kneel back on to your ankles (place a pillow under your buttocks for some extra comfort) and try leaning your upper torso forwards a little, rubbing your thighs rhythmically with your open palms in time with your breathing. Focus on the rhythm of the rub then your breath. Now rest.

IN THE ALL-FOURS POSITION

18. Sway your hips from side to side in rhythm to your music (rock away that pain). Breathe rhythmically and try the 'Aahh' sound. Focus on your sway, then the music, then your sound. Then rest.

19. Paddle or kick your feet rhythmically up and down on to two pillows. Focus on the rhythm of your kick. Now rest.

20. Beat one stress ball on the floor rhythmically while balanced on your knees and one hand. Listen to the thump sound. Count the beats in your head. Use the 'Aahh' sound over and over. Focus on the ball and then your voice. Now rest.

21. Rock and roll your hips around, then rock your body forwards and backwards. As you do so, make the 'Aahh' sound. You could also try smelling some grapefruit oil dabbed on a tissue. Focus on the movement then the sound. Now rest.

22. With a hot pack on your back, say out loud, 'Relax, relax, relax.' Focus alternately on the keyword and the heat. Now rest.

LYING DOWN

23. Lie down on your left side with a pillow between your legs and one of your stress balls in your right hand. Bang the ball on the surface in front of you. As you do so, hold a tissue scented with orange oil (or another oil of your choice) in the other hand to sniff as you please. Focus on the ball then the scent. Now rest.

24. Lie on your side (either side) with a pillow between your legs, supporting your upper leg. Close your eyes and visualise the baby turning. Say to yourself, then out loud, 'Turn, turn, turn, baby, turn.' Focus on the mantra. Now rest.

25. Lie on your side (either side) with a pillow between your legs and say, 'Aahh,' as your partner massages your lower back in circles or long sweeping strokes. Focus on the sound and the feel of the massage. Now rest.

Transition – now it gets tougher!

Just for a moment, imagine yourself in well-established labour, let's say at about 6 to 7 centimetres of dilation in the first stage. Only about 3 centimetres to go until you reach second stage! You feel great. You have done well to have come so far and have now hit transition.

The next contraction is beginning its enormous wave. You feel the power, you feel the pain, you feel your body tension and ... *you panic!* You do nothing! You freeze! What do you think the next 60 seconds will hold for you in this state?

It will hold an overwhelmingly powerfully painful sensation. It will absolutely overload you. You will be on the edge of losing it. You may have nausea (sniff spearmint oil dabbed on a tissue if you do). And you may start to feel a bit of a victim in your own labour. You will feel as though you are stuck in a trap, bombarded by pain and panic.

Sometimes transition throws at you nausea, shaking, chills, back pain, 90-second contractions with double peaks, and a premature pushing urge. A premature pushing urge does not mean you are in second stage. You are still in first stage and this may make it confusing and exasperating for you. If the baby's head at this point is not fully rotated each transition contraction will be pushing the head towards the bowel rather than the vagina. This pressure establishes a strong pushing urge, eliciting the bowel stretch receptors in exactly the same way that a second stage pushing contraction does with the lower vaginal stretch receptors. Because the urge feels the same from both places it is impossible for you to tell it is a rectal pushing urge, not a vaginal pushing urge. You will want to push, but your midwife will tell you *not* to.

This is the time you will put all your energy into panting and blowing – or yelling or crying out if necessary – and avoiding any gravity- assisted position (try getting down on all fours or lying on your side). Let your body continue the labour process until you get to full dilation. Some of you will not be able to fully control the urge to bear down. Don't be too hard on yourselves. Your overall objective here is to resist the urge to bear down to the best of your ability.

Transition has many challenges, maybe enormous challenges for you and your partner. You have to do something, and you have to do it now! But let's freeze frame for just a moment while you answer the following questions:

- Am I a resourceful human being?
- Am I healthy and informed?
- Have I been going well up until now?
- Am I curious to see if I can get even bigger than my pain?
- Am I safe and supported?
- Is my baby okay?
- Have I tried sniffing peppermint oil to freshen me up?
- Have I exhausted all my options yet?
- Am I willing to try for a bit longer?

Now it's time to get real

Transition is unpredictable – it could pass in 15 to 20 minutes! To prepare for it, pick out some of the practice ideas above and repeat them, but this time really *get bigger than the pain*, and really *turn up the dial*. Don't forget:

- Big stress needs big expression.
- Big surges of adrenalin need big actions.
- Big pain needs big rushes of endorphins.
- Big 'I can'ts' need big 'I cans'.
- If you feel stressed, do a releasing activity. *Let it out!*
- If you feel angry, breathe an angry breath, make an angry sound. *Let it go.*
- If you are frustrated, stomp with determination – it's only an emotion. *Get rid of it.*
- If you feel vulnerable, bash your stress balls to remind yourself that part of you is strong, very strong! *Bash harder.*
- If you feel scared, say so – if fear is acknowledged, it seems to lose its grip on you. *It's healthy pain.*
- If you run out of ideas ask your midwife for suggestions. *Distract yourself with her.*
- If you feel you are losing it, match the pain – big time! *Get bigger than the pain.*
- Remember you are only human – if you need help during labour, then you need help. *Talk to your midwife.*

If you find you don't have the time to physically practise, then practise in your mind, with strong active images. Don't forget to look at some photographs during practice for strong visual references. Simply going through the motions of labour practice is not enough. I want you to consider the benefits for you of these skills during labour as you explore the practice exercises. You do have some significant labour objectives to work towards:

- less pain, less fear
- shorter labour
- more endorphins
- less stress, less panic
- more control
- depletion of adrenalin
- release of more oxytocin
- working with your body
- working with your partner
- inspiring yourself with your involvement.

Sarah's top-ten tips

On page 220 you will find a list of the things you can take with you to your labour suite to help you with your birth skills. The following tips are perhaps just as important to take. These were repeated to us over and over again in class so we'd remember them. I took notes, and here are my notes for you. I hope they help.

1. Inform your doctor and midwife before you go into labour of your intention to use your birth skills and other birth plan ideas you may have for your labour.

2. Stay as quiet and as inactive as you can for as long as you can to prevent early fatigue – you just won't know how long your labour will be. Use more active, dynamic strategies only if the passive ones are not effective, and build these up slowly to match the pain. Again, don't overdo it too early as you may tire quickly.

3. If you have a medical induction of labour (an IV drip in your arm) with a sudden onset of pain, you may need to use more active, dynamic strategies almost immediately (negotiate a slower drip pace if possible). And remember, you can still move around and use the shower and bath with the IV drip.

4. If you find one or more birth skills are not working for you, put them aside until later and try something else, or just change your environment. You could try the shower, bath or spa.

5. Keep your partner informed of where the pain is – show him by putting your hands exactly where it is on your body and tell him if it changes position, otherwise he is guessing. Tell your partner also if you don't want timing, talking or to be touched.

6. If you find your birth skills moderately helpful, but falling short of your expectations, ask your partner to join in by mimicking exactly what you are doing, with the same rhythm and intensity. Together, you can step it up even more. Listen to him. Watch him. Match him.

7. If you have reached the limit of what you can do, in other words, if you have exhausted every avenue of your own resourcefulness and feel you cannot go on, do not feel a failure for needing to request assistance from your medical staff – whether that is more ideas, moral support, nitrous oxide mask, pethidine or epidural.

8. This point is obvious but is repeated often because it's true: nothing comes before the safety of mother and baby. If your doctor needs to step in and make medical decisions that affect your labour (for example, extra monitoring equipment, IV drip, epidural, vacuum extraction, caesarean, etc.) adapt your birth skills to manage the change.

9. Listen to your attending midwife for guidance; remember he or she has attended hundreds, if not thousands, of birthing couples and has a wealth of knowledge and experience in helping women through labour.

10. Stay flexible, stay open; you have incredible potential as a human being to cope with and manage childbirth.

And as an extra golden tip, remember: It's wonderful that you are giving the birth skills a try.

Sarah's labour kit bag

Here are some of the helpful items you might like to take with you into labour:

- clothes: large T-shirt, jogging bottoms, nightie, dressing gown; comfortable shoes and socks
- toiletries: face flannel, mouthwash, lip balm
- skill tools: hot packs, stress balls, cue cards with keywords, watch with second hand or stopwatch, wooden back massager, massage oils, visual aids such as pictures of Harbour Bridge
- for the shower: shower cap, swimwear for your partner
- food for your partner
- sports drink or Juju's special labour aid for sipping between contractions – 85 g (3 oz) honey, teaspoon salt, 85 ml (3 fl oz) lemon juice, 1 crushed calcium tablet, 1 litre of water (this can also be frozen as ice blocks for sucking).

By no means is this list exhaustive. Most hospitals will provide:

- beanbags, floor mattresses, fit balls
- some aromatherapy oils and electric oil burner
- showers, baths, spas
- ice blocks, hot packs and towels
- fridge and microwave.

Check with your own hospital if any of these are not available; if not, you can arrange some of them yourselves.

And finally ...

Some researchers believe that practical rehearsal, even silent mental practice, encourages the brain to send nerve impulses out to various areas of the body. Therefore the experience is not just a series of mental pictures, or a fantasy of labour. Make your labour practice as rich as you can so that when you arrive at your birth location you feel almost as though you have done it all before.

See yourself in your home or at the hospital you are attending as you practise. Smell the smells, hear the sounds, see some of the faces you know, imagine your partner right there, just as though it really was the day of the birth of your baby. Think of the mental practice Olympic athletes do. Practise with mental imagery, when you are calm and quiet and centred. Visualise the birth as if it was really happening. The practical preparation and the mental imagery are staples of training for mastery.

I hope you and your partner have had some fun together practising the skills. As this is all new for you, dealing with inhibitions is going to be a large part of the preparation process and laughter always helps with shyness. Laughing together is certainly an important part of my classes.

Now we are going to move to preparation for your labour by looking at one of the most common problematic labours: posterior backache labour. If you don't understand what it is, you will not know what to do if you have one, but more importantly you may do all the wrong things, especially use the wrong positions. May I encourage you not to skip this chapter because you think this will not happen to you ... it just might.

Posterior backache labour

You might have heard the term 'posterior labour' referred to as a 'back-ache labour'. Not all posterior labours have backache; they may have different signs. This is why you need to have some knowledge about these often very difficult births so that you can problem solve according to your own situation; you can then make any necessary adjustments to your birth skills during the contractions.

What does the term 'posterior labour' mean?

Posterior relates directly to the placement of the baby's head in the pelvis. A posterior baby is head down, but her head is the 'less than normal' way around; that is, the top of her head is in the back or posterior part of the woman's pelvis – technically, to the back-right quadrant or the back-left quadrant.

As labour begins the baby is usually positioned head down with her spine running down the inside of your abdomen, slightly to one side. Her face would be pointing towards your back. The baby's spine in this position can be felt on external abdominal palpation. The most common position is called 'LOA', which means 'left occipito anterior' – the occiput (or hard top part of the baby's head) is in the left-front part of the woman's pelvis. In this position, the pressure of the contractions moves the baby's head down on to the soft dilating cervix easily. The pressure of the hard top of her head on the cervix is good as it stimulates the labour contractions and makes them more efficient. Without this pressure, the labour would be less efficient. The occiput could, of course, also be in the front-right quadrant (ROA) of the pelvis and the cervix would receive the same pressure. The diagram below shows a baby in the anterior position.

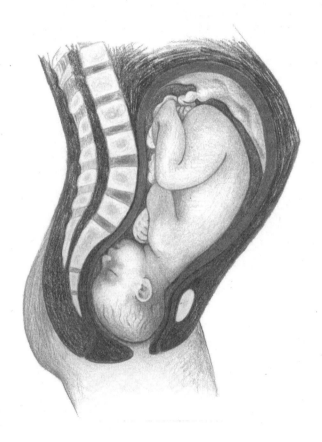

If the baby is in a posterior position then it would not be possible to palpate her spine through your abdomen as her spine would be running alongside your spine. This means (assuming the baby stays posterior during labour, though she can turn) that the pressure of your contractions can push the hard top part of her head directly on to your spine or pelvic bones or joints from the inside, thus causing you backache. (See diagram below.)

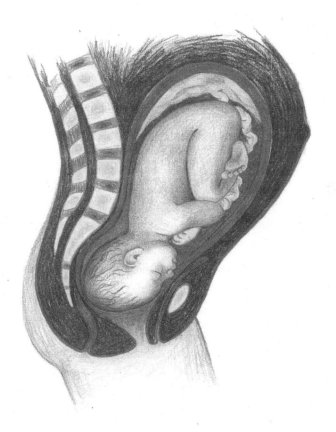

I spend a lot of time in my class demonstrating these positions with a rag doll and pelvis to make sure the positions are understood by the class members. It's a really good idea to work out these positions with your partner so you both know exactly what they mean, using a teddy bear or soft doll as a demonstration baby. You can also do this well with an old white sock. Draw a face and a navel on one side and some curls of hair and a line for the spine on the other. Turn your demonstration baby upside down and rotate her four times, as through the four quadrants of a pelvis, making sure you identify where your spine and her spine will be. You should be able to work out each quadrant of the pelvis – Front left (LOA), Front right (ROA), Back left (LOP) or Back right (ROP), these last two being posterior. It's too late in the middle of a posterior backache labour to try to comprehend these presentations of the baby in the pelvis, so make sure you understand them now.

What can I expect in posterior labour?

First off, if a baby is in a posterior position in late pregnancy it is usually of no consequence to the birth. It doesn't even mean your early contractions will turn into a long backache labour. You see, the baby might rotate back to an anterior position with the early contractions of labour. In fact, most of them do rotate at some point to the correct anterior position. Unless you actually asked your doctor or midwife to tell you of the position of the baby on the last two or three visits before the birth, you wouldn't even know the baby had ever been posterior. Some babies need to get into the pelvic inlet in a posterior position, but turn to anterior once this entrance has been navigated. Do not go into a panic if your baby is in a posterior position before labour begins. Also, if you have had a lot of backache during pregnancy, it bears no relationship to the position your baby will take in labour. So, again, don't feel anxious that you might have a long backache labour.

Unfortunately, most women hear only the 'horror stories' relating to posterior labours, and usually from women who had no knowledge about how to manage them. Well, you will know what to do.

The problems you may be faced with if your baby is in a posterior position are:

- pain in the back and, later on in labour if the baby has not rotated anterior, in the rectum
- a lack of productive pressure of the hard part of the baby's head down on to the cervix as this very important pressure pushes unproductively on the pelvic bone or spine, creating a lot of local mechanical backache that usually increases as the labour

becomes more established – this is a form of labour pain that is not meant to be there, and it is usually more intense than uterine contraction pain

- less-efficient contractions and unusually slow dilation, due to a lack of stimulus from the baby's head directly and symmetrically on to the cervix – the baby's head is pointing unproductively towards the bony pelvis instead
- irregular contractions, also due to a lack of firm and increasing symmetrical pressure of the baby's head on the cervix; some women describe the contractions as 'all over the place' – if you write down the time intervals between contractions and the duration of the contractions, you will usually find they are very different from the textbook outline of contraction patterns
- fatigue, because a posterior labour can be much longer than an anterior one – it's really important to know about this in advance because often your fatigue will start clouding your perception of everything.

'Gentle birthing' techniques may not be powerful enough to help you with the very intense posterior pain.

One interesting thing is that you will not feel the labour pain in your abdomen if you have strong back pain. It is still there but the intensity of the back pain overrides the uterine labour pain. And don't forget: *most posterior babies will turn during labour*.

What do I do during posterior labour?

Let me repeat (you know I like to): *most posterior babies will turn at some point during labour*. The ones that get stuck and never turn are only about 6 per cent of births. If you know that most will turn then why not have a go at trying to influence the rotation of your baby as early as possible. Use positions that favour the rotation of your baby in the pelvis and conversely prevent her head from further deflexion. *Don't panic, be proactive!*

Picture a soldier standing to attention. His head is proudly tilted upwards and backwards and fixed in that position. This is the picture of deflexion of a baby's head inside the pelvis when she is in a posterior position. This does not hurt the baby, but it does create a wider surface area of the baby that needs to negotiate the bony pelvis and muscular birth canal. As well, the unique moulding of the baby's head to allow a smoother passage through the vagina does not take place in this position – the moulding narrows down the surface area as the baby moves deeper into the vagina. All of these things – the posterior position of the baby, the deflexion or tilting backwards of her head, and the inability of the skull to mould well – will prevent her achieving a snug fit in the pelvis. This will contribute to problems with dilation, rotation and descent.

The positions you can use to help the baby turn will be the all fours, the stand–lean, side lying, and crouch kneeling with your back parallel to the floor. Do these only during contractions. In between you can rest. You can even have this break in an upright position if you want to, but as soon as the contraction returns, resume one of your posterior birthing positions. *Do not*: stand up, walk around, bounce on a fit ball or sit astride a chair until your midwife confirms your baby has rotated to the anterior position. *Remember: Don't panic, be proactive.*

By using your posterior positions and avoiding gravity, your baby's head will drop away a little from the spine, possibly decreasing backache, as well as achieving a little contact with the cervix. Your partner can assist you with the backache by applying deep massage – long sweeping pressure over your sacrum – rolling a wooden back roller in all directions over your back, putting hot packs over the area of pain, and sometimes applying hard pressure with his elbows or thumbs right down into the dimple in your back. Remember: *Don't panic, be proactive.*

You are also going to help yourself with all of the skills and tools you have learnt from the previous chapters. Distraction will be especially important for you at this point as the pain of a posterior labour is not healthy pain! Stress balls, vocalisation, heat, showers (lean over a plastic chair), oil on a tissue, music, and any movement that blocks the pain will all be part of your plan. This plan could also include banging the floor mattress with a stress ball or your open hand, rocking your hips from side to side – furiously kicking your feet up and down on the floor mattress and rocking forwards and backwards as you are draped forwards over a fit ball in the all-fours position. Your keywords and visualisations will be focused on 'Turn baby'. *Don't panic, be proactive.*

You are also going to communicate more often with your doctor and midwives. It is important to listen to their wise counsel about any medical help you might need. Many women struggle through posterior labours, eventually having an epidural when they can bear the pain no longer. This can mean that they have all feeling blocked out for second stage when they need to help the uterus push out the baby. Sometimes it is preferable to discuss the use of an epidural a little earlier rather than later. After an epidural the baby often turns as the mother relaxes, then the epidural wears off and the woman can push out her baby with normal sensation. There is no guarantee but it does happen.

Sometimes, when struggling with the contractions for a long time, the baby's head can become more deflexed and what might have been a posterior labour with a good outcome becomes a more difficult posterior, needing even more intervention. I am not suggesting you have an epidural, and I am not suggesting you don't have an epidural, I am not suggesting you have one early or late, but I want you to be aware that with a posterior birth the decision for an epidural is not based solely on your tolerance of mastering labour pain; it has so much more to do with the position of the baby's head, the ease with which it can turn, and when it will turn.

Above all else: *Don't panic, be proactive.*

What about before labour begins?

- Many of the women in my classes ask me what they can do before labour to prevent a posterior labour. Well, other than exercise, stretching, back mobility workouts (especially if you have a sway back), and good luck, there is not much. The position of the baby is largely dependent on the size and shape of the pelvis and the size and shape of the baby's head. No matter how much yoga, swimming, walking or floor scrubbing (this one is an old wives' tale!) we do, we cannot change these two things. As well, it is thought there may be a correlation with the placenta being on the anterior wall of the uterus, a sway back in the mother, an overdue baby and a woman over 35. These are only correlations, not causes, so don't go into a spin if you are 38 and having your first baby. I will say again, they are only correlations and *most posterior babies turn at some point in labour!*

- Two studies, one in Canada and one in Sydney, both showed that activities in the all-fours position in late pregnancy demonstrated no detectable difference between groups of women who did it and those who did not. My feeling is that it is best to wait until the contractions start and then, and only then, start to use your turning postures to correct the baby's position. This will minimise your fatigue and boredom with the positions. It is not until the uterine contractions start to warm up that the muscular fibres have any influence on the baby. The uterine musculature has three sets of fibres that all fire off simultaneously under the effect of oxytocin. There are fibres that pull the cervix open, there are fibres that press the baby downwards into the pelvis, and there are fibres that exert a torsional pressure on the baby. These are the fibres that are responsible for turning the baby. With a baby in a posterior position, these fibres will work most efficiently when you are in an all-fours position but only in the presence of a contraction.

Labour begins at home

The first thing you are going to do when your labour starts is to ask yourself the posterior questions. These are:

- Do I have backache (sometimes not present)?
- Where is the backache – is there any rectal pressure?

- Are the contractions irregular? (Remember to record them.)
- Did my midwife or doctor tell me my baby was posterior in late pregnancy?
- Where were most of the baby's movements yesterday – in the front of my abdomen?
- If I lean over (the kitchen bench, for example) does the back pain remain? (This could mean you have a simple anterior labour with some referred pain in the low back – phew!)
- If this is your second birth, was the first birth posterior? (It could be a pelvic disproportion situation – the size and the shape of baby's head in relation to the size and the shape of pelvis.)

If you answered yes to two or three of the above questions then you need to work out what to do to facilitate rotation of the baby's head as early as possible. If you are convinced your baby is facing the 'wrong' way, then you will need to start your positional work early in labour to have the greatest effect in preventing extra deflexion of the baby's head. This hopefully will help an uncomplicated posterior remain an uncomplicated posterior. Even if you answered no to all the questions above, I encourage you to check again and keep checking throughout your labour, especially if backache or a slowing of dilation occurs.

Write down your answers so you can accurately report all this information to your midwife when you call the hospital. If you are not sure if the baby is posterior or anterior when you are still at home, use the posterior positions anyway. Your midwife on admission will confirm the baby's position and then you can immediately change your positions to more upright ones if necessary.

When it is time to leave for the hospital, adjust your position in the car so that you are as comfortable as possible. Make sure you have a hot pack for your back. With my second baby I stayed at home for nine hours, thinking that this was best. On arrival I was only 1 centimetre dilated! On reflection, I should have gone in sooner to be assessed by the midwife as I was using all the wrong positions at home and I was creating a greater deflexion of my baby's head – it turned out to be a very long and difficult posterior birth. Keep in touch with your midwives by phone, and listen to their advice.

The trick (well, it's not a trick at all, really) is to: *Ask, ask, ask, ask, ask, ask, ask, ask, ask!* If you don't ask the medical staff and you don't know the position of the baby you may make the mistake of using the wrong positions, making a simple posterior a more difficult posterior. This could lead to a more complicated delivery, possibly a caesarean. If your midwife says she is not sure at the time of admission of the position of the baby, then at least avoid activities such as bouncing on the fit ball or pacing the floor for long periods until the next examination. Use movements like gentle body swaying while you are leaning over a bed, table, bench, or sink. Further on in the labour if it becomes clear that the baby is posterior (maybe by now you realise the dilation is slow, you could have had an early pushing urge or rectal pressure, back pain is increasing, contractions are irregular, the baby is not descending at all), then simply progress to a more forward-leaning position in which your back is parallel to the floor. If the examination confirms the baby is in the right position, then you are free to explore the full range of gravity-assisted positions for the first stage – standing, bouncing, walking upright, kneeling, etc. If the baby is in the posterior position try to influence the rotation of the head as early as possible.

Will labour slow down if posterior positions are used when the baby is anterior?

Maybe a little bit, but the positions are worth doing if you are not sure. Once you arrive at the birth location and are examined by the midwife and the baby is anterior, you can make up for lost ground by really applying yourself to the contractions, encouraging the baby's head on to the cervix, using gravity to help your baby down into the pelvis, rocking, swaying, walking, bouncing gently on the fit ball, letting the pain out, working off the adrenalin, and letting your oxytocin flow. Oh! And don't forget to get your endorphins flowing!

What can my partner do to help?

If the baby remains in a posterior position your partner's work will be cut out for him. He needs to stay as refreshed as possible. Make sure food is packed for him – he will need the energy. As the contractions become more and more established, the backache usually gets more intense, and he will be attending to you with every contraction, to help you get through it. He may get tired, frustrated, despondent, disappointed. There may be times when he is filled with feelings of hopelessness and helplessness and the physical exhaustion has taken all the excitement out of labour. He just wants it over. These are normal feelings. Morale can drop for him too.

His mantras for you will not include 'Healthy pain', because posterior pain is not healthy pain. He will need to focus more on 'Pain out', 'Stress out', 'Baby's turning'. He needs to keep checking your positions. Remind him *most posterior babies turn at some time during labour.*

If your baby doesn't turn and you need to have the nitrous oxide mask, pethidine, epidural, forceps or vacuum extraction in the second stage, or maybe even a caesarean, your partner needs to know he did brilliantly, he needs to know that no one could have done any better than him as a support person in the same situation. The last thing anyone wants is for either of you to feel a failure because you were not able to conquer this extremely difficult birth using only your own resources. (I had two posteriors and I didn't conquer either, but I still gave birth and I still have two beautiful children!) We do the best we can in life with all the experiences we are thrown into. With education, insight, a positive attitude and a little luck, we are able to make the most of everything – even a difficult posterior birth.

You must know my philosophy by now: equip yourselves and give it a try! But also have plan B and plan C at the ready in case you need them. By no means do I want to sound like Pollyanna but it was because I had those two very difficult posterior births with my own children that I changed the course of my physiotherapy career. Two easy births would never have ignited in me the challenge to make it a better experience for others. It became a drive and a passion to do so. I don't know what I would have done professionally for the last 30 years otherwise, but I would never have had the gift of meeting so many incredible doctors, midwives, women and men in the childbirth arena and my private practice – the backbone of my daily work. It is also the reason I never let my women go into labour without being fully educated on the topic of posterior labour, and why I have included a chapter on it in our book.

Massage techniques for your partner

You might as well take advantage here! Some good movements are:

- long, slow strokes
- large or small circles
- thumb pressure
- fist pressure
- hand squeezing.

You can use oil or powder, hot or cold packs and wooden rollers.

A good lesson

I want you to read a letter from Lara, a woman from my class. It is a shortened version of the very delightful one she sent to me after the birth of her first (posterior) child.

LARA *Dear Juju, I want to tell you about the birth of Cooper. Everything you said about childbirth was true! You can't plan it, it hurts like hell, and it is the most wonderful experience you can ever go through. Ever!*

While my labour was long and incredibly painful, we were fully prepared and ready for whatever came our way. Because it was such a long labour, I think we used nearly every skill you taught us. I guess I should start at the beginning.

I was induced 11 days early as I had been diagnosed with late onset gestational diabetes at 34 weeks. My baby was big for dates. Two hours after the application of the prostaglandin gel I was in cracking labour! Contractions were coming about every five minutes and I started to use the stress balls to help with the pain. My husband started counting in a one-two-three-four rhythm. As you said, this could end up irritating me after a while and it did, so I had him change to five-six-seven-eight … Aahh, much better!

After two hours of using stress balls, I added the 'Aahh' sound throughout the contractions. I then moved on to techno music (don't ask me why) and started moving in time to the dull 'doof doof' beat in the background. It worked until I remembered my years of nightclubbing, then I felt ill! While [I was] repeating, 'Baby down, baby down,' and remembering to turn my pink oxytocin tap on visually in my mind during contractions, my husband was applying the most heavenly massage to the incredible pain in my lower back.

Next I tried aromatherapy oil on a tissue and I have to say the lemony citrus smell got me through some of the worst contractions throughout the night.

By 2 a.m. I was having contractions one minute apart, but felt they were still bearable, so I jumped into the bath with my trashy girly book, my stress balls and my ice cold face flannels and attempted to read in between contractions, crushing my stress balls on the side of the bath to distract me from the back pain each time a contraction came. I did this for the next six hours.

By 8 a.m. I was in considerable pain and I was getting tired. My obstetrician wanted me out of the bath so that he could examine me and maybe break my waters to get things moving a little. Getting from the bath to the bed seemed, at the time, like running a 50-kilometre marathon. The back pain was excruciating, although I had little or no abdominal pain. The contractions were now 30 seconds apart.

After the doctor broke my waters the pain got even worse. Then he delivered the final blow: 'Lara, the baby's head is posterior and you are only 1 centimetre dilated.' Can you imagine how I felt? All I could think of was, 'Where's my lavender oil Juju said would calm me down, before I smash something!' One centimetre! One centimetre!

On the positive side, my obstetrician was very impressed I had done 12 hours of pretty tough labour with a posterior baby, including six hours of contractions just one minute apart. Thank goodness for your posterior class!

By this time I was in serious pain. It was then that I chose to take a vote, in between the worst contractions ever, asking everyone in the room if they thought I was a wimp if I had an epidural. Everyone's reply was, 'Of course not!' To me at that point it was the only option as there was no way that stress balls, massage, lemon oil and vocalisation were going to get me through another 12 hours. No one had any idea just how long I had to go. Within seconds I was ordering every midwife that could hear me to get the anaesthetist on the phone to tell him I would pay double if he got there in 10 minutes! Four minutes later he was there.

The moment the epidural went in I almost divorced my husband and proposed to the anaesthetist! I could have kissed him! Such incredible relief. In a much more relaxed state, even having a bit of a sleep, I dilated to 10 centimetres in two hours. My obstetrician was brilliant and came to check on me countless times.

Finally it was time to push. I told the midwives I knew how to push using the coffee plunger technique. I thought about that coffee plunger for the next two hours. Eventually the baby's head crowned and I asked my obstetrician if we could try to get him out without an episiotomy. He agreed but said it might take a little longer as the baby was big. Then he began perineal massage and I watched with a mirror the miracle of my baby's head presenting at the vaginal outlet, and then coming out. Quietly and calmly, at 4.14 p.m. my 3.7-kilogram baby boy was born. I had a minor graze internally (requiring three stitches) and two hours later I was up and showering.

I can honestly say that despite experiencing the worst pain I have ever felt, over the 22-hour period, I would do it all over again tomorrow. Childbirth was the most magical experience ever. My labour was far from perfect but I did it and coped with it, my way.

There is so much to learn from Lara's story: one human being's ability to cope with pain; what limitations there might be; how a team of people can support the labouring woman; the listening, feeling, caring professionals that are there to help; how joint decisions can be made when the team works together; the loving support of her partner. Lara's second birth was also a posterior labour, but much, much better. She said it was a totally different birth except for the excruciating backache. It was only five hours, with an epidural at 8 centimetres, a great second stage with three gentle pushes and no stitches. The second time round, Lara's husband even delivered their second beautiful baby boy!

And finally ...

If you have never experienced a posterior labour, you can wonder what all the fuss is about. You probably think, 'Well, don't all labours have excruciating pain?' Yes, they certainly have very, very strong pain and pressure, but these sensations are only from the uterine muscle working and the pain is 'healthy pain'. With posterior pain there is a pressure from the bone on the baby's head pressing on the bone of the woman's pelvis and it is 'unhealthy pain'. This is the difference.

Sometimes a baby is in a very simple posterior position and the woman breaks all the rules and manages to have a quick natural birth. This could apply to you, but please be prepared in case it does not. As with any labour, take a posterior labour contraction by contraction, applying your birth skills as you go. Your positions are paramount, right from the beginning. And if the back pain gets totally out of hand and you need some or every bit of medical assistance available, see it all as part of the incredible adventure of the birth of your baby, with your choices, your way.

The posterior backache labour chapter is a little 'heavy' but I would not have included it unless it was absolutely essential. *Knowledge is power*, especially if you have a posterior birth. I hope you now can begin to ponder the likelihood of such a labour before the birth, identify the signs early, start your action plan long before you arrive at your birth location, apply the correct strategies, know the questions to ask your midwife, be involved with her and your doctor in appropriate problem-solving decisions, hold on to your feelings of empowerment even though a shared decision may result in medication or surgery, and to remember that birth is all about having a healthy baby.

It is only natural now that the next chapter introduces you to some medical and surgical choices and some of their other indications for use besides posterior backache labours. You may choose intervention through simple preference, or because of an emotion such as fear, or a physical state such as fatigue, or an inability to deal with the pain. On the other hand you may experience a medical complication when you will be presented with options to choose from. In case of an emergency any decision making may be taken out of your hands, and your professional team will take immediate action.

I have chosen stories that are inspirational, not because I want everyone to choose a medicalised birth, but I want you to think about how you can contribute to making the birth of your baby as positive an experience as possible if you do need drugs or surgery. Too often I have seen women who have had a drug-free birth say joyfully, 'Wow, I had a natural birth!' and women who have had an epidural or caesarean birth say despairingly, 'I had the works!' It shouldn't be like this. Childbirth is joyful no matter what. The following detailed accounts of birth with intervention from women in my classes say it all.

PREPARATION

Medical help if you need it

I hear, over and over again, that women are not helped by reading or hearing disappointing or negative stories about childbirth. I'm a great believer in making education for childbirth real. Occasionally, women who have been at my classes take a long time to process their birth experience. This can be from the disappointment of having to have a medicalised birth, a long posterior backache birth, a birth that progresses too quickly or a birth that they felt totally out of control with on all levels.

Everyone has a story to tell about their labour. I have chosen to include in this book some epidural and caesarean stories from women in my classes, not just because they are so positive, but because they are inspiring as well. This book focuses on the human resources each woman has to enable her to master childbirth. Sometimes, however, it will not be possible to have a totally natural childbirth. Dealing with a medicalised birth is beyond the intended scope of *Birth Skills*, but familiarising yourself with some stories of women's experiences with epidural and caesarean births may enhance your understanding of both. All of these women came to my classes. Each wanted a natural birth with no intervention, and they worked hard towards that goal. On the day, however, things turned out unexpectedly.

Women who have had only natural births often cannot understand why others may need or choose medical assistance. This puts tremendous pressure on those women who do. Read these stories carefully; they carry their own wisdom, challenge and joy, and may give you a greater appreciation of the wonder of birth, however it happens.

Meredith had a birth using the birth skills, medical induction, an epidural and a caesarean. The reason for this medical intervention was pelvic disproportion – the baby's head was too large for her pelvis. Her story begins opposite.

Possible reasons for caesareans

- Failure of labour to progress.
- The baby's head is too large for the woman's pelvis.
- Maternal or foetal distress.
- Placenta praevia, when the placenta is abnormally low, lying over the cervix.
- Abruptio placenta, when the placenta separates prematurely from the wall of the uterus.
- Prolapsed cord, when the umbilical cord comes through the cervix and vagina before the baby.
- Active maternal herpes.
- Transverse lie of the baby.
- Some difficult posterior presentations.
- Some breech or multiple pregnancies.
- High maternal blood pressure.

Possible reasons for an epidural

- Pain relief.
- To lower high blood pressure.
- Maternal exhaustion.
- A drawn-out birth with posterior presentation.
- For caesarean birth.

MEREDITH *Our baby was due on 27 December but did not arrive. We agreed to an induction if I had not gone into labour by 6 January. I was praying this would not happen but I went into hospital on the night of the 5th and was given the ripening gel at 9 p.m. I took some sleeping tablets to get some rest so my husband went home, expecting to return around 8 a.m. the next day when my waters would be broken and a syntocinon drip [a synthetic oxytocin that initiates, maintains and augments contractions] inserted. Thankfully, the contractions started spontaneously at 3.30 a.m. – yeah!*

Because of the tablets, I slept in between the contractions for a while. My husband arrived at about 4.30 a.m. It was the natural, slow, steady start that I'd really wanted and all I needed for the pain was a baby rattle (a modification of your stress ball class) for that soft shaker distraction and some good slow release breathing, adding a hanky to my nose with some mandarin oil to sniff.

My second support team member, a good friend, arrived at 7 a.m. and by that time I really needed both her and my husband. For around 14 hours the three of us laboured Juju-style. My husband shook shakers in my ears the entire time, starting with the rattle, then moving to a cute pink gift box with rice in it and finally the Tic Tacs (more creative ideas to focus on from class), which became the longest-enduring item. I started banging the stress balls together soon after my friend arrived. I knew they were going to work for me because I had been so convinced of their effectiveness when we did the squatting exercise in class.

The three of us were vocalising our lungs out the entire time. Lots of 'Aahhs'. My husband encouraged me by saying, 'Great releasing, Memee.' Both my support people were amazing. Quite amazing! It really felt like the three of us were in labour. This shared the burden in a most extraordinary way. My friend would 'Aahh' louder than me most of the time and she'd change the rhythm or the sounds we were making, going from 'Aahh, aahh' to 'Aahh, eehh, ee, oh, ooo' and back again. I really had to concentrate hard! This was fantastic as it kept me focused. We spent some time in the shower too and that was great. I'd lean on my husband and my girlfriend would direct the water to the hurting parts, while I kept banging the balls.

At 12 noon, 'we' were 7 centimetres and our baby girl was progressing so well. Moving down, doing all the right things and showing no signs of distress whatsoever. So on we went. The staff shift changed and the midwife that came in said, 'You must be a Juju girl – no one chants like that unless they've been to Juju's classes.' The midwives at my hospital were great incidentally; totally supportive of us being as vocal and mobile as we needed.

The crushing blow came at 4.30 p.m. People kept asking me if I felt the urge to push and I really wanted to say, 'Yes,' but I just didn't! They did another internal and I was still 7 centimetres (double damn it!) It really was crushing. My baby was lying transverse and not moving anywhere in a hurry. At this point the contractions were full on, really intense, coming right on top of each other and lasting up to two minutes each … relentless!

When the obstetrician said she wanted to augment the labour I knew I couldn't carry on. I'd reached my breaking point and I couldn't cope with it getting any more intense than it was. I asked for an epidural. I asked my husband if he'd be disappointed and the look on his face was priceless. I knew that he'd never been prouder of me than he was at that moment.

After the epidural was inserted I lay down and went to sleep for I don't know how long. They hooked up the syntocinon and in that time our baby turned and I dilated fully to 10 centimetres; the rest was just what we both needed. The great thing was that the epidural had worn off enough for me to feel and push.

We pushed for around an hour, with my husband encouraging me to think coffee plunger and my girlfriend telling me I was making the most of every contraction – mind you, the midwife had to keep reminding them to not bear down with me or they'd give themselves haemorrhoids! The obstetrician and wonderful midwife were happy with how we were going but then the baby started butting up against my pelvis, which apparently was too small for her to squeeze through. Later too, once she was born, they realised that her big, hard head was part of the problem too – it was not going to mould to squeeze through and it had started to swell up. We didn't know that at the time so it was a trial of forceps for me, which quickly proved to be an inadequate solution. We were taken into the theatre for a caesar. Phew!

It was such an interesting (not sure that's the right word?) experience, going through all the above decisions. I thought the C-word would be the end of the world for me but it really wasn't. Same with the augmentation and the epidural. It was all just the way it had to be in the end. My husband and friend were unreal at supporting every decision I made and my obstetrician was amazing – I never felt pressured to do things one way or another and she never once made the situation sound like a dire emergency. At each turn, I felt like I was presented with the options and all the facts so that I could be a major part of the decision-making process. So that was good. I never felt like I lost my power in the situation.

At 9 p.m. (exactly 24 hours after the process began) our daughter was born! She was the most perfect, beautiful creature I had ever seen and I couldn't have cared less how she came out. I was a blubbering mess, and so was my husband. The caesar was a bit annoying but there is no way I would have traded the 14 or so hours of labour we did for going straight to the operating table. It was an incredible experience and I feel really thankful for that. I feel like I could do anything now. I feel like my husband and I could do anything together. Plus, I think labouring naturally for a while released lots of the right chemical stuff and it meant that our daughter fed as soon as they brought her up to me at *midnight! I was so thankful for this because it was one of the things I wouldn't have wanted to miss out on.*

It's funny now looking at my birth plan and how much of it did not go according to expectations. I still just feel so grateful for the experience and don't regret any of the things that happened in the course of those hours. Our daughter was born safe and healthy and beautiful and I survived relatively unscathed.

It was such an empowering experience and so enriching to go for it and give my all (with my amazing labour team) to the process of birthing my daughter. It was an incredibly exhilarating time and I know that there are things that have been irrevocably changed in me as a result, making me a stronger person, a better partner to my husband and a freer, better-equipped mum to our beautiful daughter.

Childbirth is not a competition, nor is it about a plan. It is a wonderful journey involving you, your partner, your support team, your professional birth team and, of course, your baby. When everyone is working as one dedicated unit, your birth will be fabulous, just as Meredith's was. I find her story honest, heartfelt, human and above all inspirational.

Annie had an epidural due to pain, exhaustion, and a posterior presentation.

ANNIE *Well maybe it was Murphy's Law but I had a posterior labour with an epidural. Despite this I have extremely warm and wondrous memories of the labour and birth of my baby. I was just so moved spiritually by the whole process. It was wonderful and exciting, and my husband and I are amazed at how quickly and totally we fell in love with our baby.*

I was 1 to 2 centimetres dilated on the last visit to my obstetrician. Over the next few days nothing much happened. My obstetrician knew how much I wanted to try for a normal vaginal delivery without drugs or an epidural if possible, so we agreed to hold back an induction for as long as possible. But 11 days after my due date I was admitted to hospital in the early evening and given the first application of the gel to try to induce the labour gently. Both my doctor and the two midwives who admitted me said they thought the baby was in a posterior position. They asked if I knew what that was and of course I replied, 'Yes.' They were amazing and kept me informed of everything.

Two hours later 'bang', the first contraction came. The midwife ran the bath for us and I got in on my hands and knees (I took the foam you suggested for my knees and ankles). I started rocking on my hands and knees, sniffing lavender oil from a flannel, and repeating over and over, 'Turn, turn, turn.' My husband set up the stereo and generally made our delivery suite room like home. I had a beanbag, a floor mattress, various height chairs and stools, stress balls, essential oils, different coloured flannels for different oils, music ranging from schmooze to jazz, rock, classical and opera. I used everything.

Just after midnight I started to develop serious back pain. I moved from the bath to the floor mattress, and started using the stress balls as my main pain-management tool. I banged them against the wall, floor, mattress and together. I also started to use vocalisation – loud vocalisation – in order to block the pain. I then changed my position to standing leaning forward over the delivery bed. This made it easier for my husband and my second support person to apply the hot packs and provide massage over my back with the wooden rollers.

By 3 a.m. I was dilated to 5 centimetres, but I was getting tired and the back pain was massive. The midwife was there always making new suggestions and brought me the gas first with the mask and then with the mouthpiece so that I could bite on it if it helped. It didn't. By now I had everything working together: hot and cold packs, massage, sound, stamping, stress balls, visualisation, music, and rocking sideways vigorously. My second support person and midwife were coaching me as well. Then the midwife picked up a second set of stress balls and banged them with me and used eye-to-eye contact as the music got louder. My husband was trying to count, but as the contractions were irregular (another sign of posterior) this became quite difficult.

My next examination showed the cervix was 6 centimetres dilated. I was by now exhausted. I knew I could not go on, I had given it my all, and I needed help. I decided to have an epidural.

The anaesthetist was fantastic and very calming. As well as explaining everything he was doing, he also commented on the tools I was using. Both he and the midwife were impressed with all my 'aids' and also that I had gone this far without help. Once the epidural took, I had total pain relief, but also chills, shaking, teeth chattering and got freezing cold, but blissful pain relief.

My obstetrician arrived at full dilation to tell me the baby was still posterior, but had descended. An hour later the baby had rotated somewhat and I could feel the pushing contractions. I was elated. Pushing down felt very powerful. My midwife kept telling me to push into my bottom.

After another hour without much progress my doctor suggested the option of assisting the rotation with forceps. I had everyone around me doing different things – giving me oil to sniff, spraying my face, giving me ice cubes, encouraging me to push, brushing my hair, all with my Maria Callas' 'Madame Butterfly' at full blast. Our baby came out with the forceps and three pushes. He weighed 3.5 kilograms and I had only two stitches for a small episiotomy.

I'll never forget how I felt when he was placed on my abdomen. It must be the best feeling ever. I couldn't believe how big and perfect he was, and believe it or not, I could have had the birth all over again. I felt powerful and informed, cherished and respected by all those around me. Everyone was there to help and support me. The circumstances of the birth were more difficult than I had *anticipated but we did it – we all did it. It was an incredible experience with my husband, my friend, the midwives, the anaesthetist and the obstetrician. I look back on it with great joy.*

Annie, you had the perfect use of epidural – as backup when your own resources could take you no further. The fact that it wore off as you needed to push out your baby was a bonus. In some births it is difficult to decipher where the rewards of the mother end and the rewards of the support people begin. I suppose it's just all one big achievement of the maternal team with the mother at the centre. I can't help but wonder Annie, as your beautiful baby was being born, if it was 'Un Bel Di' ('One Fine Day') that Maria Callas was singing? Surely the whole experience was earth moving! I can see it all and feel it all. Congratulations!

Julie, whose story follows, had an elective caesarean birth because her baby was breech.

JULIE *As you know I was positively anticipating the birth of our daughter. I was 43 years old and had been trying to get pregnant for years. We (including my obstetrician) regarded the whole event as miraculous.*

At the 36-week scan the baby was in a perfect position with her head three-fifths engaged and nicely placed in an anterior position. At the 38-week visit my obstetrician could no longer feel her head. After a quick scan we found that she had moved into a breech position, and that there was now a cord presentation over the cervix. This meant that if I went into labour without her changing position again, an emergency caesarean would have to be given.

Not wanting to be involved in an emergency situation, I elected to have her delivered by caesarean section with an epidural block at nearly 39 weeks of gestation. As it turned out the elective caesarean turned out to be a good decision as she had turned again into an even worse position. Just goes to show, best laid plans ...

I'm feeling fine about the whole thing and am just incredibly thankful to be able to hold a perfectly formed little human being in my arms – something which I had begun to think would not be possible.

Julie, your birth experience also reminds us all that sometimes in life we have to change our plans and intentions. Having a plan B or plan C as backups in your mind is essential. Openness is essential. Flexibility is essential. As I read your story, I have renewed appreciation for both informed choice and modern medicine.

The next report is by Lucy, who started her labour using birth skills but needed an epidural and caesarean as full dilation did not progress.

LUCY *I always thought I would be the type of person who arrived at hospital in labour and immediately asked for an epidural. I changed my mind. After years of trying to fall pregnant and much disappointment I now wanted to experience everything. At my first birth skills class I was quite struck by comments from some of the second and third timers who had returned to refresh their knowledge for their new births. They described their labours as awesome! I thought the classes might help but I couldn't imagine myself describing labour as such.*

As the classes progressed it all started making sense to me. I had recently completed a psychology degree and your explanations of the psychology and neurochemistry accorded with my own knowledge. Knowing I don't like surprises, I wanted to be prepared. The knowledge was calming for me and I felt I could be in control.

I had been sharing what I had learnt at each class with my husband, who was a little sceptical but willing to let me do this my way. After the partners' class, we talked about what we would do and how we would manage labour. I bought a project book and he bought a stopwatch. Together we compiled our labour kit, which included the essentials, like my labour book, stress balls, lollies, stopwatch, heat pack, lavender oil. The entire kit cost about 40 Australian dollars (the stopwatch was about 30 dollars).

In my labour book I had summarised the key messages from classes. The first page of the book had all the hospital details. Pages two and three had the words 'relax' and 'release' in big purple letters. Pages four and five had a beautiful picture of the Harbour Bridge (from a calendar) and the words 'open', 'down', 'turn' in big letters. The subsequent pages had other keywords and phrases – 'lock it in', 'coffee plunger', 'healthy pain', and even the names we had selected for our baby, just in case I forgot what all this was about!

Labour began late in the afternoon. I had a 'show' [release of the mucous plug from the cervix] just as we were about to go to my parents for dinner. During the evening I was feeling more uncomfortable – I could feel the tightening of my uterus – but no pain. On the way home the contractions were becoming more regular and we were so excited. At home we got the labour kit ready and called the hospital. The midwife told us to come to the hospital when we felt ready.

The contractions started coming harder and faster. My husband was timing them and I was marching around the house 'Aahhing' and breathing in my lavender oil. I set myself little goals to make the time pass. At 10.30 p.m. I promised myself a shower at 2.30 a.m., but not before. Just after we rang the hospital again. It was time to go!

During the car journey I was banging the centre console with a stress ball for distraction. I was 4 centimetres on the initial examination. We set up the room with the stereo, my book and the stress balls. My husband was fantastic. He was keeping time, telling me to get ready and counting me through each contraction. He would remind me to 'match' the intensity of the pain and suggest different tools if he thought I was struggling to maintain control.

At 4.30 a.m. I got into the shower with the showerhead angled at my back (where most of my pain was). When the contraction started I would march and splash the water with my feet and 'Aahhed'. As the morning progressed I was dilating steadily and the midwife told me it wouldn't be long, but it started to slow down. To try to move things along I decided to have the membranes ruptured. Finally about midday the midwife told me I could start pushing.

I was feeling ready for anything at this stage. I had got through the first stage of labour and felt very powerful. Well, I pushed and I pushed, but nothing happened. Pushing was harder than I had imagined, but I was working on getting the technique right and trying to make each push effective. I tried pushing in every position – lying on the bed, squatting on the bed, squatting at the end of the bed, sitting on the birth stool – but after two hours, the baby had not moved. I was getting tired and frustrated and the doctor ran through the options: keep pushing, suction, forceps or caesarean. He felt a caesarean would probably be inevitable. The baby was coping but the doctor was getting concerned.

Our objective going into labour was the safe delivery of our beautiful baby, so after another 30 minutes of unproductive pushing, a decision was made for a caesarean. Once that decision was made it was all systems go and 10 minutes later we were in the operating theatre. At 2.45 p.m. our beautiful baby, a healthy 3.7 kilogram boy, was born, just on 12 hours after we arrived at the hospital.

Having said at the outset that I couldn't believe women described labour as awesome I am now one of those people. Labour was the most awesome experience of my life. I loved every moment of it: I loved the control I had over the experience and I loved being able to share it with my husband. In my mind it was a great team effort.

My doctor asked me later in the day if I felt disappointed about having a caesarean. I said 'no'. Going into labour, I had one objective: the safe delivery *of our baby. I felt great pride and satisfaction in getting as far as I did. I had a rich birthing experience (yes, 10 minutes of that were surgical) and can honestly say it was the best 24 hours of my life. I can't wait to do it again!*

Lucy, you did indeed have a rich birthing experience. When you and your husband visited my classes to report your birth, your effervescence, pride and joy was overwhelming. I forever will remember and re-quote what you said about it being the best 24 hours of your life, and of which 10 minutes were surgical! I know many women who had a similar experience, except they focus negatively on the 10 minutes of surgery rather than the 23.5 hours of adventure!

Vicki used birth skills at first and then chose an epidural before having a caesarean due to high maternal temperature and failure to progress.

VICKI *I had a very healthy baby boy, and even though I ended up having an epidural and caesarean birth, I have no regrets. Did I want an epidural? No. Did I want a caesarean? No. I went into labour with a wealth of knowledge and understanding and therefore understood the reasons for the outcome and felt empowered by the decisions I made during the birth.*

My waters broke with no contractions on Saturday night. On advice from the hospital we went in. Unfortunately, I had a temperature when we arrived so I was closely monitored. My contractions started at midnight and by 7 a.m. were regularly five minutes apart. By 10 a.m. they were two minutes apart and lasting 60 seconds. On examination I was 5 centimetres dilated and all seemed to be going well.

I was coping with the pain by applying heat packs, rocking, hand rubbing, and later leaning against the basin while I stamped my feet. My husband was using a wooden massage tool on my back and I added a stress ball and vocalisation as the pain built even more. This was all working well. Due to the fact that I had to lean horizontally because of severe back pain I strongly suspected my baby was posterior, but at this stage I was confident the baby would turn and all would be okay.

By 1 p.m., with increasing severity of pain and consistent two-minute contractions, I was re-examined and found not to have dilated any further. At this stage I suspected I could be in for a very long and arduous labour with no guarantees that he would turn. So after 13 hours of labour and looking at an indefinite amount of time ahead of me, I began to look at the pain-relief options.

I tried the gas for a few hours, which helped with the pain but not the dilation. I decided to have an epidural but even so, for five hours I had strong and fast contractions but had dilated only one more centimetre. The result was a joint decision to have a caesarean. My temperature had started to rise again and I believe I could have been there another 10 or so hours with only a small chance at the end of having a natural birth.

Before going into labour, my aim was to have a natural vaginal delivery. I did not want a caesarean, but that's just the way things go. I feel really positive about the experience because I know that if labour had progressed normally and I had continued to dilate, the strategies you taught me would have seen me through to a natural birth. I am very confident I would have endured the pain and coped for significantly longer if things were progressing. I also know that if I had not had the understanding of the process, I possibly would have felt like I had done something wrong, had failed and been very disappointed. As it is, I see it as one of those things that happen and I am even more confident about having another go at natural birth the next time.

Vicki, well done. You will take to your next birth a belief in yourself, a sense of being empowered by what you did in this birth and the courage, confidence and knowledge to give it another try. This is what birth (and life) is all about. It is often the women who feel they have failed or done something wrong who start out their parenting days with feelings of failure and despair after blaming themselves, or sometimes blaming the medical staff, for a situation that was beyond their control.

The difficulty with childbirth is that before you actually go through it, it is a fantasy, and as a conscious, creative creature you can put any story into that fantasy that suits you. Then comes the reality! And much that you can control, and much that you can't!

Vicki's story carries adult and conscious decision making, and an insight for us into the lessons in life from which wisdom is made. Vicki was absolutely right: it was 'just one of those things that happen'. Getting the experience into perspective is a wise lesson for all of us.

Our next story comes from Juanita, who used the birth skills and then had an epidural and emergency caesarean because she was overdue, the baby was large, sitting high and not descending, then foetal distress developed.

JUANITA *Our big baby boy is thriving and although we didn't have the natural birth that we had hoped for, he arrived safely, and for that we are grateful and happy.*

Hang out the sign that says, 'Abandon all your expectations!' All our plans for a natural water birth at the hospital were well in place. We had our bag of tricks packed and my husband had written a list of what to say and do. As the due date came and went we started to be a little concerned that the perfect birth was not progressing as it was meant to.

After two weeks the hospital midwives suggested we see an obstetrician. He advised us to have an induction in two days' time. We were still determined to have no medical intervention, so the day before the induction was scheduled I had two sessions of acupuncture to bring on labour. Labour pains started that night and by 5 a.m. the next morning I was having regular contractions.

Feeling like we had everything under control, we headed off to the hospital at 9 a.m. On arrival, I was a bit disappointed to find I was only 2 centimetres dilated. Nonetheless, the contractions felt quite intense and I soon found that the fit ball and the hot pack were my favourite tools. I bounced up and down on the ball and bashed the stress balls together. My husband timed the contractions and we were amazed to see that they did, indeed, last for exactly one minute. As the contractions got closer together, I leaned over the wooden dresser and swayed my hips from side to side. My husband banged the stress balls together for me and told me to 'See yellow, see yellow'. I also found it helped if he counted me down through the contractions so I knew how much longer I had to go. I found the counting and rhythm enormously helpful in managing the pain. I also vocalised right from the start, matching the pain as it got more intense.

After about four hours I moved into the shower and spent the next couple of hours in there. The hot water pressure on my front and back was a fantastic relief. I had been drinking chilled sports drinks, but as the contractions got more intense I started throwing that up, so we stuck to water.

We were very disappointed that after 12 hours of labour I was still only 3 to 4 centimetres dilated. The midwife suggested she break my waters. At that point all hell broke loose! I finally understood what you meant when you said the pain can be colossal! Suddenly there was wave upon wave of the most overpowering contractions. I got back in the shower and we ran the bath, but I found myself not coping as well because there didn't seem to be any rest period between contractions; the pain seemed constant.

It was the one thing I hadn't been prepared for. I kept saying, 'There's no rest period! Where's the rest period?' With no down time in between contractions it became harder to focus on the techniques. I remembered the chart from classes that showed the early contractions as smooth waves, and then how they progressed to high jagged peaks – that's exactly what it was like.

All the time, my husband was amazing. I am still so impressed with his strength and courage. Thanks to his calm demeanour I didn't for one second feel any panic or concern. It made all the difference in the world. We were even cracking jokes and having 'normal' conversations about mundane things, which was quite bizarre.

Without any real rest periods in between contractions I was finding it hard to gather my strength and use the skills I had learnt. My vocalising was the last thing I lost control of. When I couldn't control my 'Aahhs' any longer, I finally asked for pethidine and gas. I struggled on for another four hours or so, moving between the bath and the beanbag.

When the midwife checked me again I was still only 4 to 5 centimetres dilated. For some reason the baby was not moving down. At this point I said I didn't think I could do it any more. The midwife said she felt I could continue for another four hours or so without intervention but my husband said he felt I was genuinely exhausted and unable to cope any longer. If I had been 8 or 9 centimetres I would have kept going without a second thought, but I had a feeling things were not going as they should.

After 16 hours of labour, I had an epidural. I have to say, when the drugs kicked in and removed the feeling of pain, it was the most blissful relief of my life. Unfortunately the baby went into distress and I ended up having an emergency caesarean, which just goes to show you should never get too attached to your plans! I had worked very hard to have a natural birth and I felt

I was well prepared but, with all the goodwill in the world, in the end it simply wasn't possible.

Our baby was enormous – 4.5 kilograms! – and the doctor said he wasn't pressing on the cervix because his shoulders were wedged against the pelvic bones and they were taking all his weight and holding him back from descending. This made sense. Both the doctor and the midwife agreed that with his size and positioning, I probably could never have given birth naturally.

People have said to me, 'Oh what a shame, you had to go through 16 hours of pain; you may as well have just had the caesar straight up.' Strange as it sounds, I loved the whole experience – I am so pleased I experienced those 16 hours. So to anyone who says, 'Well what's the point of going through labour if you end up having a caesarean?' I would say that the labour is the point. It is the biggest experience you will ever have in your life and I am so grateful I went through it.

Without the coping techniques, I know I could not have persisted for so long. Childbirth certainly presents women with the greatest challenge they will ever face in their lives. Whether they make it only part of the way, or all the way, it doesn't really matter. The important thing is that we honour this precious gift we have for giving birth, and giving life to another human being. I now have a real sense of respect and wonder for what our bodies are capable of, whereas before I might have just seen it as a yukky, painful process to be got through as quickly as possible with the help of lots of anaesthetic. I am in awe of the whole process, and it is without doubt the greatest experience of my life.

Juanita, I have read your story many times over the last two years; it has been shared with many women – thank you. Each time I read it I see and learn new things. I could not have written this chapter without your story because above all it has 'intelligence' written all over it. Intelligent plans and preparation. Intelligent choices and attitudes. Intelligent reflections upon it. As the sophisticated and intelligent race of people we have become, I see no other way to be.

Now Melissa used her intelligence as well and elected to have a caesarean with a spinal block because she had high blood pressure and her baby was sitting high in the pelvis.

MELISSA *Having gone to all your classes during pregnancy and being confident and psyched up for a natural birth, to be told at 40 weeks I might need a caesarean quite shocked me. I remember feeling such mixed emotions and tears when I walked out of the doctor's office.*

The baby had not moved down nor engaged into my pelvis. My blood pressure had risen and remained higher than it should have been. My doctor believed that if there was no movement or contractions in the next four days then a caesarean was the safest option for myself and my baby. My doctor was not forceful in any way and I did trust his advice. Four days later the baby still had not moved. I talked it over with my husband and we decided we should have the baby delivered by caesarean. We were booked in for the next morning.

It was a bizarre feeling driving to the hospital that day, knowing that I would have a baby by the end of it. I was a little apprehensive that it was all so planned. I was also disappointed that it was happening this way as I thought the operation would take away some of the special moments I had been looking forward to. I didn't want it to be sterile and impersonal. I couldn't have been more wrong.

As they wheeled me into the operating theatre my nervousness was immense. My emotions were all mixed up about what was about to happen. The anaesthetist was brilliant – so calming and even cracking a joke to calm me down. The spinal block went in without a hitch and I didn't feel a thing. The nurses were so friendly, my doctor was so positive. And I had my husband by my side and my cousin was there as well.

We all felt ready ... it was just a change of location. My husband sat just behind my head at one side and held my hand. The screen was up and the operation began. And guess what? Even having a caesarean I used my knowledge from classes. It didn't go to waste. While I didn't need the more active techniques, I focused totally on my husband's face and didn't think of what was going on below. I didn't even hear what he was saying, I just focused on his face and eyes.

Just when it was getting to the point when the baby would emerge, I unlocked my focus and turned my head to the screen. One minute later, the doctor lifted my screaming baby over the screen. It was a boy! My husband and I reached out to touch his little hands. It was the most amazing moment I have ever experienced! I started to cry, overwhelmed with emotion.

After the cord was cut my cousin took some very special shots of the three of us. While I had always wanted a natural birth, my baby would not have come out naturally due to his position – the doctor confirmed this.

The birth was just as amazing, just as special and just as memorable, and we have a gorgeous, happy, healthy boy.

Melissa, I have just re-read your story as our book goes to print and all I can say is I have tears in my eyes at the emotion, celebration and joy that I feel from being privy to the birth of your baby. I then had to remind myself that it was a surgical birth. But that's the whole point, isn't it? The baby is gorgeous, you are both safe, the birth was amazing, and we can feel your emotion and be deeply moved by it. What a powerful message.

Adrianne faced the possibility of a caesarean birth but learnt her birth skills just in case she needed them. And she did use them, as well as gas and an epidural as pain and stress relief in late first stage.

ADRIANNE *Even though I was hopeful of a natural birth, I was considered 'highly probable' for a caesarean as I had a grade 4 placenta praevia (the placenta covering the cervix). An ultrasound at 35 weeks showed the placenta had moved from the opening, which meant we could try for a natural birth.*

At 37.5 weeks my waters broke at 4 a.m. With excitement and a slightly surreal feeling, my husband and I headed up to the hospital with our labour kit. For the first five hours the contractions were like minor cramps and were easily manageable (my husband amused me by passing the time juggling the stress balls!) Not expecting anything to happen soon we went for a walk around the hospital and watched a baby bathing class. A short while after this, active labour suddenly started and we headed back to the labour suite. It was very intense with contractions coming between 30 seconds to one and half minutes apart, with each contraction lasting around 90 seconds. I stepped up my coping strategies utilising swaying, humming tunes, squeezing a stress ball and using the shower on my back and abdomen.

My husband was not able to count me into the contractions because they were so variable. There was just no rhythm to them. However, he did a fantastic job bringing me water and encouraging me with positive statements like, 'You are doing really well, honey,' and 'The baby is coming down.'

I was doing well, but decided to try the gas to take the edge off the intense contractions. I found that the gas restricted my breathing and my ability to vocalise through the contraction. I persisted for about 30 minutes, but my coping strategies were well and truly disrupted. By the time I requested an epidural I was 8 centimetres dilated and very happy with my progress.

I was given a single 'blocking' epidural rather than a continuous one. The epidural did not hurt at all when it was administered (there was a slight pressure on the lower back) and it allowed us to relax for an hour. The labour was progressing very quickly. Due to the lightness of the epidural I was able to feel the contractions; but they were not painful.

At full dilation I was able to start pushing. It was wonderfully empowering to be able to feel the contraction and push down using your [Juju's] coffee plunger imagery. After 45 minutes of pushing the baby's head was just visible, but due to the baby's rising heart rate, the doctor decided to give an episiotomy and use the vacuum to assist with delivery.

Looking back on the birth, I have such positive feelings because throughout the whole pregnancy I was told I would probably have to have a caesarean and although I ended up having medical intervention it was still a vaginal delivery. If I could have that birth again, I would not try the gas, as it was the turning point for me towards not coping. I realise the gas works wonders for many women but for me it was the wrong choice.

I feel very proud of myself as I worked through the labour with all my birth skills up until 8 centimetres and then helped to push out my baby. Even though I have a little regret that I picked up that gas, I certainly have no feelings of disappointment about the epidural. The whole experience was an incredible achievement for both of us.

Adrianne, don't be too hard on your decision to try the gas. You are right, it works well for many women: you weren't to know it would interrupt the flow of your pain management, rather than help it. We will never know if you would have made it through that birth without medical intervention and, in a way, it just doesn't matter now. You worked wonderfully with your husband and you have your beautiful healthy baby.

Harriet had an epidural about two hours into second stage labour because there was no progress after two hours of pushing.

HARRIET *I wanted to tell you [Juju] that the birth skills I learned with you were fantastic. I dilated to 9 centimetres in about five hours, dealing with the pain and moving the whole time. My main tool for the pain was using the stress balls, and I used them every way possible – on the wall, on the bed, on the floor, against each other. My husband had his own pair and spent most of the time pressing them into my back during the contractions to help with the back pain. Occasionally I used a bit of nitrous oxide gas but I found that the 'Aahh' sound was actually more effective than the gas.*

I made a point of relaxing in between each contraction, as my husband did any running around necessary. We were very excited when the midwife told us, 'It won't be long now,' as she started getting everything ready for the birth. She told me to start pushing when I felt like it.

As I started pushing I could visualise my baby in my arms and this gave me tremendous motivation to push with all my might. But nothing happened.

I pushed for about two hours with no progress. The baby was stuck and I just could not bring him down. The obstetrician arrived and tried to help deliver the baby with vacuum extraction, but eventually it was decided I would need forceps with epidural.

I had a drip, a catheter, constant monitoring, and then the forceps. Thanks to the skill of my obstetrician I avoided a caesarean and our daughter arrived healthy and without a mark and I was still able to help push out my baby with the epidural.

Even though the delivery was not exactly how I planned, I did find the whole experience a positive and empowering one. The first stage was brilliant and we used most of the techniques you taught us. I could do it all over again. I went into it feeling informed, powerful and strong with lots of pain mastery techniques at my disposal. I was amazed at how uninhibited I was (at one point I was squatting stark naked over the squatting bars), and I was given every chance to have a natural birth. The mental strength and positive attitude I gained from giving birth have flowed over into this time after, at home with my baby.

I know how much you wanted to have a completely natural birth, Harriet, but in your situation, an epidural was called for. I remember immediately after the birth you told me you were a little disappointed about this, but by the time you wrote this letter to me I see much of the processing of that disappointment has been accomplished. For your next labour you want to have a natural birth and are certainly working towards that in my classes but, as I always say, let's work towards what is possible, but be open to plan B and plan C just in case.

And finally ...

As human beings, we get out of bed each morning and live each day as positively as we can. We do not say to ourselves, 'Now, I must live this day as negatively as possible.' For that reason, I have included stories here with only a positive edge to them, to encourage any of you who need or choose an induction or epidural or caesarean to also be able to seek the most positive experience possible, even though you may have set your heart on something different. If a medical choice is made at some point in your labour, be proud of what you have done up until that moment.

Childbirth is not like the Olympics in which the top three athletes in the world get the prizes and the recognition. In childbirth, we all get the prize, and we all get the recognition. Every birth is important, every birth is special – if for no other reason than it heralds the beginning of new human life. This is a celebration in itself! Perhaps the journey of a medicalised birth is the most inspiring as there are more hurdles to jump, more difficult decisions to make, and more challenging and persistent feelings to work through afterwards. Once birth is behind you and you are busy parenting, the process of giving birth gradually becomes like a speck in the ocean. You do not lose, or fail, if your birth is not whatever you saw as 'perfect'. You gain your baby, you gain experience and you gain wisdom from getting through a part of your life that is much, much bigger than yourself.

Cherish the birth, it is precious no matter what, and write it down when you get a chance, because one day, probably when you are least expecting it, you are going to be asked, 'Mum, what was it like giving birth to me?' Then you will have that inspiring story to tell!

Motivation and psychological strength – especially courage, confidence, determination, certainty and the ability to step beyond perceived social sets of rules – in labour are a large part of what my classes are about. You need to bring the physical (your birth skills) and psychological (your mental and emotional beliefs and attitudes) together in order to harness every bit of inner strength you have. And then use it! I find this such an exciting concept and I delight in hearing every day the stories from couples about how they motivated themselves through extremely challenging circumstances. Ultimately the pride and sense of achievement they feel as a result puts them in good stead for the all-important parenting of their child.

Researchers say that our willingness to step beyond our limited beliefs about what is possible enables us to master the motivation to action, which is what we are discussing next.

PREPARATION

Motivation and birth skills

Mastering labour pain is exciting but not easy. Coping with labour pain does not seem to be related to pain thresholds, fitness levels, alternative exercise activities, educational degrees (or lack of them) or occupations, your mother's or sisters' births, your nutritional behaviours or any other factor you might like to suggest. I might also inform you that being a knowledgeable health professional also does not help. Of course, many of these things may contribute to assisting you to manage labour, but do not rely upon them as the answer to or the guarantee for an easy birth.

I wish I had a penny for every time a woman said to me, 'The pregnancy has gone really well so I'm expecting the labour to be smooth and proceed with no problems.' It's just not that simple; it's a false correlation. Perfect pregnancy does not mean perfect birth! The great news is, though, we are all on an even playing field when we have a baby. It means that coping with labour is not reserved for a select group who may, for example, swim, attend yoga or tai chi classes, read lots of birth books or attend multiple sets of antenatal classes. A major contributor towards your ability to manage your pain is the belief system you have about yourself and your ability to cope. This is where insight and knowledge comes in. Another contributor is the intrinsic drive you have to give it a try. This may be conscious or unconscious, but it will be there. Sometimes, though, it is hidden beneath the fear.

Proactivity, possibility and potential

Human beings respond to challenges; we love to discover what we are capable of. We have an innate drive towards exploration. Some more than others, but we all have the innate ability in life to give experiences a try. Even so, I have done many things in my life, but I will never bungee jump, base jump, climb Mount Everest or become a pilot. I will never commodore a submarine, an aircraft carrier or a spaceship. I might like to but, hey, we can't do everything! But I will continue to explore many other avenues for the rest of my life.

Childbirth presents us with an opportunity to pioneer the inner frontiers of humanity itself, our inner Mount Everest ascent, our own inner space expedition. What follows are some of the reasons women and men give when talking about their aspirations of giving birth as normally as possible. These reasons drive them towards their goals. They give them the determination that they need to take on the challenge of childbirth. There are no reasons that are right or wrong, better or worse; they are just reasons:

- to avoid drugs if possible
- to experience the rite of passage of birth
- the emotional challenge
- the physical or intellectual challenge
- the spiritual experience
- a general sense of achievement
- the belief that birth is a natural process
- the desire to feel proud of oneself
- to use innate skills
- curiosity, intrigue and fascination about the birth process
- for an adventure
- to use their human potential
- the control of an uncontrollable activity
- for personal development

- a sense of worth
- a connection to baby and a connection to partner
- a sense of empowerment
- fear
- meaning

and many, many more. No one can tell you what your reasons may be: only you know those, but you may need to motivate yourself beyond just a set of ideas and hopes.

Motivation is all about stimulating that part of your brain that seeks higher goals (this is how collectively as a planet, 'we' put man on the moon), that desires maximisation of human potential, that strives for competence and excellence. This does not mean you must have the competence and excellence to have a perfect birth. It is all about intrinsically assisting and empowering yourself to take on the adventure of childbirth, and the experience that you are given, rather than just handing yourself and your experience over to others. It's about being self-reliant.

Think about it this way ...

We are all told so often that we are given so many special gifts in life, but we do not even bother to take off the wrapping and look inside. What if childbirth was a little like that beloved game we all played at children's birthday parties – usually the last and most important activity of the day. Do you remember sitting in a circle, the music playing, your little heart beating, and the very beautiful parcel making its journey around the circle? When it came to you, did the beating of your heart turn into a pounding? As you reached out to take it, did you do so with great excitement, anticipation? Then you held it – oh, didn't it feel so good to hold it; it felt like it was yours – but then you had to pass it on even though you wanted to hold it just a little bit longer. You'd do everything humanly possible to hang on to it until the very last second and then, just as you passed it on, the music stopped! The next child got to open the wrapping. Then the music started all over again, and did your little heart start fluttering once more as the whole process began all over again?

What if you could look at labour in a similar way? What if you could approach each contraction as one 60-second round of Pass the Parcel? Yes, naturally, there would be hope and anticipation, and anxiety and fear, and joy, and involvement, and maybe disappointment, but also the resilience to start all over again and face the music of the next contraction.

Did you read Martine's story in the chapter on breathing and vocalising? She was a little hesitant about the sound she was making to cope with the pain. And her midwife told her it was a beautiful sound, a musical sound, the sound of a woman in labour. Are you too filled with too much fear to give it a try, to take off some ribbon and the wrapping?

We also seem to have a powerful motivating force to excel when presented with an opportunity of great meaning. Most of the time women cannot identify why they wish to take on the rite of passage of childbirth – often they are responding to an internal creative drive, mostly subconscious. It seems probable that it is also part of our collective survival instinct. How clever we are to have this to help drive us forward towards the challenge that otherwise we would attempt, at all costs, to avoid.

Ten ways to motivate yourself

In preparing for your adventure these ideas might inspire you to tap into your incredible potential.

1. Think about what would drive you towards a richer and more rewarding childbirth experience. Write this down and think about it each day. **Empowerment means taking action**.

2. Remember to keep your goals, expectations and options realistic. Avoid performance anxiety – it is not an exam and there are safety nets if you need them. **Empowerment means taking action**.

3. Identify the number of weeks you have been avoiding the topic of

pain. The pain of labour is part of you, you actually create it, it's healthy pain and it is harder to fight it than to master it. *True!* **Empowerment means taking action**.

4. See yourself as being proactive in labour, not passive; see yourself as being powerful not panicky. As one of my women said recently to me, 'I just had to get gutsy, and this was new for me, but I knew with the intensity of the pain, it was either get gutsy or go under!' **Empowerment means taking action**.

5. Identify with other women's success stories to inspire and motivate you. Be sure to read all the labour excerpts in this book and picture yourself in their stories. Pain is unpredictable, so are the mechanisms to manage it. No one knows the best techniques for them until the day. **Empowerment means taking action**.

6. Learn more and more about your own protective biochemistry. Read all you can about endorphins, and although you can never see your own pain-reducing chemicals, you can increase your belief in them. You will not be alone with the pain. You will have these tiny, yet potent polypeptide molecules to help you. **Empowerment means taking action**.

7. Each time you have a shower, practise for labour. The objective is to have new habits for when you feel pain but, more importantly, you need to feel comfortable and uninhibited with these new habits. Angelina, a delightful woman from my classes, used to say that 'Although the skills make sense, if you haven't had a baby before, you may think they don't match the venue of a hospital.' Whenever she said this, other women in the class who had been through childbirth before used to answer, 'Maybe not, but they [the skills] are better than the pain!' And then everyone would laugh and nod in agreement. **Empowerment means taking action**.

8. Attend couples antenatal classes and with the help of instruction, charts, pictures, videos, discussion, etc., learn everything there is to know about the labour process and its variations. **Empowerment means taking action**.

9. Prepare yourself physically with swimming, walking, gym classes, cross training, yoga, Pilates, tai chi, meditation, weights, or any activity you prefer. **Empowerment means taking action**.
10. Repeat your own affirmations that reinforce your own limitless capacity to do in labour all that you are capable of. Have an objective of truly astounding yourself! **Empowerment means taking action**.

What's your objective here?

There is no pass or fail when having a baby. The primary objective is to have a healthy baby and a happy family as you embark on the next stage of parenthood. Your only motivating force may be that you simply wish to give it a go because 'Women have been having babies for thousands of years'. This is wonderful This is enough. Even if you are half-hearted about it all, trying is reward, contribution is reward, involvement is reward, effort is reward.

You have learned some incredibly useful responses in this book. You may safely and with confidence take it contraction by contraction, taking your adventure of birth as far as you want to. I have heard Sarah say many times that if she had not come to the birth skills classes, she probably would have chosen a very early epidural and missed out on the adventure of a lifetime. Now, as you know, she had an epidural very late in labour for a mechanical problem with the baby descending, but it didn't mean she and her husband didn't have the most incredible experience labouring and birthing their baby.

I have said before, and I'm repeating it because I believe it, childbirth is not about having an epidural, needing a caesarean or succeeding in having a natural childbirth. It is about having an adventure of a lifetime. And for some of you it will include an epidural or a caesarean. Read Lucy's story in the previous chapter: it's truly inspirational!

Sadly, some of the greatest resentment after childbirth comes from women and men who were too rigid in their birth plan and aimed unrealistically high. Trying to be perfect only disempowers you. Closing your mind to the unexpected disempowers you. Maybe approach it the other way. Have no expectations and, a bit like Pass the Parcel, just have curiosity and excitement; enjoy this miraculous experience for its own sake, and be in awe of the new life you have created.

Above all else ...

- Drop your inhibitions.
- Don't think of the last contraction, or the next one, just the one that's happening now.
- Don't worry about losing control – you may, and so what? Rest in between contractions.
- Concentrate on the task at hand, focus on your particular skill.
- Try to keep your head in sync with your body.
- It is not a competition, it's not about winning or losing, it's just 'experiencing'.
- Forget 'perfect' – just do your best.
- Don't think whole birth, just think this 60 seconds.
- Talk to your partner.
- Talk to your birth team.

Take lessons from others

I remember watching a television interview with Rex Pemberton, the youngest man ever to climb Mount Everest. The interviewer, Andrew Denton, asked, 'How did you face the fear and challenge, particularly when it all seemed insurmountable?' Pemberton thought for a moment, then replied, 'You have a sense of adrenalin, you always focus on what you have to do. Adrenalin drives you into this focus and the activity that will help you.'

Spot on!

Every labouring woman has this potential too. This adrenalin rush is not just for those clinging for life on the side of an icy mountain. Motivation is, in a way, already inside you in the form of adrenalin. That's right, a simple chemical that we all have! If you ever wondered while reading this book why Sarah and I have talked so much about adrenalin, now you know! Let's go over it one last time.

At the beginning of each painful contraction your fight/flight reflex produces a surge of adrenalin. Its function is to drive you forward both to the activity you need to do to help yourself manage the pain over the next 60 seconds *and* into the focus you need to have so that your mind does not get tangled up with the negative thoughts and judgements about the pain. Pretty darn clever, don't you think?

I love listening to the stories of the famous Australian high-altitude base jumpers, Dr Glenn Singleman and his wife Heather Swan. They appeared on ABC's 'Australian Story' and the interview centred on their 2006 world record for base jumping off Mount Meru in India (highest exit-point base jump). Now keep in mind it took six years to prepare for this one free-fall jump – 6,600 metres in 40 seconds with speeds up to 180 kilometres per hour! And Heather had never been skydiving or climbed a mountain when she started the project in 1999! Incredible!

The jump in itself was inspirational, it had been their ultimate goal, but it was some of their quiet conversation during the interview that grabbed my attention. Glenn looked pensive as he talked about standing on that exit point and finding a space in which he was so absorbed by the task at hand that fear was replaced with calm, and time stood still. He stated, 'Only by overcoming fear can you achieve your deepest human potential.'

Now there's a lesson for all of us, and it is particularly relevant for childbirth. Glenn talked passionately about the 'rush', the 'elation', the 'wow' factor, and Heather added that it was 'magic', 'wonderful', 'inde-scribable', 'the best experience she had ever had besides giving birth to her children'.

Childbirth gives us the opportunity for those same emotions – fortunately we don't have to prepare for six years, we don't have to take such incredible risks, and we don't have to jump off mountains. The elation, the joy, the magic, the indescribable feeling and the ultimate happiness can be similar, albeit in a different setting. I hear these words from the women and men in my classes all the time; in fact, it is these reports that inspire me to continue my work.

All things are possible. Effort brings reward. Think of giving it a try.

An advertising campaign for the 2006 Commonwealth Games held in Melbourne went something like this:

... there are no guarantees, no shortcuts to greatness, but that doesn't stop people trying!

My feelings exactly!

And finally ...

You are two adults working with your birth team to ensure the safe delivery of your new baby.

As the birth comes to an end so the next phase begins. The baby has now left the womb, and so has completed his or her physical birth, but individuation in life is not achieved unless this little human being can begin and conquer his or her psychological birth. The physical birth may have taken many hours but the psychological birth will take many years. Most of us are still on that journey! These are the precious years of parenting. Good luck with your adventure of childbirth and your willingness to 'give it a try', and congratulations on becoming parents and a wonderful new family.

I would like my dear friend and physio colleague Margaret Shaw to have the last word in this chapter. In her book, *On Becoming a Family: The first three years*, she says:

Parenthood is as old as life itself. It is the task of reproducing one's own kind and nurturing offspring to adulthood. Human beings are not born once-and-for-all on the day their mothers give birth to them, but life obliges them over and over again to give birth to themselves.

In the next chapter, the most beautiful chapter of all, Sarah will reinforce what's important here and show you the bigger picture.

AND FINALLY ...

The bigger picture

Finally, seven weeks after my obstetrician, Keith Hartman, suggested I attend Juju's classes, I called her. I had kept meeting women who had taken her classes and they all told me how wonderful she was, and how incredibly informative her classes are. When I did phone Juju she instantly began asking me how I felt about labour and what I knew about it. Most of my answers were, 'I don't know,' even though I must have read almost every book there was on the subject! The problem was I was so overwhelmed with information by this stage that none of the detail had actually sunk in. In retrospect the books didn't give me any practical applications for labour either, or any real idea about what I was going to experience during the birth. Juju's methods proved to be enormously practical. She provides women with the knowledge to understand birth pain, what it is, where it comes from, and the tools to help them master that pain and make informed choices about their labour. In doing so, fear, the most crippling, overpowering aspect of labour, can be controlled.

I believe we are afraid of giving birth because labour pain is the great 'unspoken'. When I was pregnant I hated that look in the eyes of those women who had been through labour. It was a look that told of an experience so awful it could not be talked about. There were also looks of pity; of knowing something terrible was about to happen to me. No wonder we're all frightened of giving birth! I firmly believe the fear of giving birth exists only because we don't fully understand what the pain is and what exactly we are about to experience. Juju's principle is simple: know what your body is doing and what your baby is doing and you will be empowered.

This struck home for me. If the women of the twenty-first century enjoy the ability to be educated about everything, why do we go into birth having no idea about what to expect? Yes, I am the type of person who reads up on everything I can. If I do not understand something, I go out and learn about it. I had tried to educate myself about labour, so why did I still not truly understand where the pain was, what it was like and, more importantly, how to cope with it when I spoke to Juju?

I began my pregnancy wanting an epidural, afraid of the pain, and wanting it over as quickly as possible. By the time I gave birth to my son, the experience I had was life-changing. Giving birth was an adventure. I don't think I can nominate anything that could compare with it for me. Okay, so I haven't climbed Mount Everest or sky-dived, but I think I have had a pretty adventurous life. But even my husband, who has climbed some pretty high peaks and has sky-dived, would tell you that the birth of our son was his greatest adventure. For us, nothing compares to the utterly fulfilling, challenging, life-altering adventure that we experienced at that moment.

Now, you may be reading this thinking, 'Yeah yeah, right. Sarah had the perfect birth. Woop-de-doo.' But if you have had a chance to read all the other women's birth reports in this book you will see I am not alone in saying how wonderful our births were for us. There are women in Juju's classes as I type this who are learning her methods, and there are women who are giving birth right now using them. I am sure if you asked them how their labour and birth was, their stories would be similar. And their husbands' would be too. Just think, it was only a generation ago that partners weren't allowed into the birthing room. Not only was this incredibly difficult for the woman giving birth, but the partner missed out on so much.

I was nervous about my husband being part of the private lesson we had with Juju. I know how some men are when it comes to labour and these classes – not many of them want to do them. Just as I feared, my husband kept looking at his watch as Juju was explaining labour to us. He was trying to look interested but I had a feeling he wanted this class over with as quickly as possible, especially when the graphic photos of women in labour came out! And when Juju had me up and stomping my feet, pacing the room, acting as if I was in labour, my husband looked at me, thinking, I thought, it was a little weird. He was probably thinking, 'This is so silly.' After Juju left I asked if he understood what we were going to do during the labour. He said he did but I doubted it.

I couldn't have been more wrong. My husband understood every bit of Juju's techniques. He took in absolutely everything we studied that night. From the beginning he started timing. It was quite funny really because when he started timing me, my contractions hardly hurt at all and I was drinking a cup of tea, having a giggle, but he kept timing! And he did so for 16 hours – non-stop. He worked with me through every single contraction. Never once did he falter. He was my rock. I couldn't have done it without him. He completely took on board Juju's methods, to the point where if he could see I was tired from moving he was the one who would add in the stress balls, or vocalisation, or whatever, to give me a change. Even though I was doing the physical work, he was there with me mentally, 100 per cent. *We gave birth to our son.*

Today we are so fortunate to have choices. We can have 10 people in the delivery room with us if we so desire. Hey, we can even video it for the whole family! What is important though, and what I keep harking back to, is this power of choice. How you choose to give birth is entirely up to you. What liberation! When people asked me after Kalan was born how the experience was I didn't have that look of pity, of the 'unspoken horror'. I would say it was incredible, powerful, amazing, wonderful. They would look back at me in disbelief! These were not the words they usually heard to describe labour. I would also say it was incredibly hard work and exhausting but it brought my husband and me closer than we have ever been. We had a real sense of accomplishment, together.

I didn't have a drug-free birth as I opted for an epidural towards the end. Do I feel like I failed? Not in the slightest. Our birthing experience was ours and wherever it took us was just right. It is so important to remember – and this is what I love about Juju as she constantly reiterates this – there is no failure. However you give birth remember it is your birth, your way of doing it. Juju just wants to give women and their partners the opportunity to understand their bodies, to understand labour, and to make informed choices about their pain management. There is no right or wrong. There are no good or bad choices. Except, perhaps, the choice not to learn.

My labour started at 11 p.m., so I really hadn't slept much before then. From that moment, though, I was calm and ready. Excited even. Not once, and I promise you, not once was I scared. I never had a moment of doubt about whether I could handle it. I felt great, empowered and ready – bring it on! How many other women could say the same? Initially I had very light contractions, a pinching feeling right in my abdomen. I could draw a small circle around the pain; it was isolated to an area about 10 centimetres in diameter. I thought maybe it was false labour as it was still four days before my due date. But I got out my books and read that I should start moving around straight away; if the pain ceased or got lighter then it was not real labour. So I just walked around the bedroom for an hour or so and the level of the pain very slowly increased.

The hospital had told me to call if my contractions were five minutes apart but I was already ahead of that. My contractions were four minutes apart from the start! As they were only mild I waited a while and didn't call my obstetrician until about 1.30 a.m. He told me to relax for another hour or so but to call him if I couldn't talk through the contractions. My husband was asleep at this point so I woke him up and said, 'I think this is it!' We were so excited. He immediately got out his watch and started his timing! In between contractions we both had our showers and checked I had everything in my labour bag ... and we waited.

As I waited I lay on the bed, breathing slowly, or leaned over a chair. I tried to do as little as possible as I remember Juju saying to save the big guns for when the pain gets big so as to not tire myself out. Keith, my obstetrician, called me about an hour later and asked if I would like to go to the hospital. I still thought that maybe I wasn't really in labour so I hesitated but then decided I would rather get there just in case it was the real thing. I figured I could always go home if it wasn't.

Juju taught us a lot about labouring in confined places; that is, in the car, in a lift, even in the hospital reception! I was lucky that my contractions were relatively painless. As my husband and I drove to the hospital I remembered the stories of other women who had to bang their stress balls and use sound during their journey to the hospital. I remember the husbands in Juju's classes talking about their panicked driving, jumping red lights. Well, my husband decided to play it safe and we cruised to the hospital averaging 30 miles per hour, chatting and laughing the whole way! This certainly wasn't like the movies!

We arrived at the hospital and Keith came in to check me. I was 3 centimetres dilated and hadn't really felt a thing! Piece of cake, I thought. My mum arrived a short time after and as the contractions increased I walked around the labour room, had cups of tea and biscuits, and chatted happily. My midwife, June, kept coming into the room to get me moving – she knew I had a long road ahead of me even if I thought it was pretty easy. Plus, the best way to keep the labour progressing was to keep active.

Keith had predicted the baby would be born by 9 a.m. so he didn't come back to see me until about 6.30 a.m. Even though I had been walking around the room and keeping active, when he checked me I had progressed to only around 5 centimetres. Keith suggested breaking my waters to speed things up and we agreed. Wow! It certainly did speed up ... the pain!

As the contractions became stronger I used all the different birth skills I had learnt in Juju's classes. As I sat on a fit ball and rocked back and forth while leaning against the bed my husband continued to time each contraction, preparing me for the next one, talking me through the pain by using visualisation, and encouraging me to use sound. After a while my midwife suggested I move into the bath for a change. I agreed as I had heard how the wonderful weightlessness provided by the water can reduce the pain, and I guess at this point any change was welcomed as I was getting tired. With every step from the fit ball to the bathroom I was counting on this working as the pain was increasing exponentially – at this stage I was now 7 centimetres dilated.

Unfortunately, the bath made me feel queasy so I opted to go back to the fit ball, rocking and making 'Uh-uh' sounds, focusing on the sound of my voice and the inflections it made. Then my husband handed me the stress balls and

I banged them together for about 30 minutes. I concentrated on the colours and on the sound they made. They were fantastic but I was tired and my arms started to ache. It was at this point I wondered whether to get an epidural.

It is incredible how quickly you can switch off the self-control and confidence. As soon as I questioned whether to give up, the pain got bigger than me. It was a terrible feeling so I began to focus again and I was soon back in control. I kept myself strong, I kept in control. I cannot stress how important that was. Keith checked me again: I was 9^1/$_2$ centimetres. I would say this was the peak of my labour, and it was definitely the most trying as it required intense concentration.

My contractions were now all on top of one another and it was tough to distract myself from the pain and to focus on my techniques. It was difficult for my husband to time my contractions as there seemed to be no beginning, middle or end. At this point he moved on to just coaching me through the contractions. He worked with me through the pain, encouraging me, helping me. He kept me focused on the positive: I am giving birth, my baby is working his way out, it is healthy pain, I am nearly there.

My midwife kept checking to see if I felt the urge to push. I didn't. Keith came in to see me again at about 10 a.m. and told me the baby had pushed his chin upwards and had created a lip on my cervix, stopping him from coming down. I was stuck in transition! This was a real test of my concentration and stamina. Having had no sleep all night I was really exhausted. Keith, my husband and I decided it would be best for me and the baby to take the epidural. Even though I was almost there, just another half a centimetre, it would help me relax and bring the baby down.

It takes quite a long time for an epidural to be set up – about 15 minutes for the anaesthetist to arrive, 15 minutes for the equipment to be set up, and about 15 minutes for it to take effect – so I needed my birth skills during this time more than ever. I kept using sound and visualisation, hanging on to my husband through each contraction. Our faces were about 20 centimetres apart as we kept going through it together. Slowly I got relief from the epidural and we were able to be quiet and to relax. My throat was hoarse from using sound.

After about an hour Keith checked me again and the baby was right down and ready to be born. The epidural hadn't worn off so we waited another hour but I still couldn't feel anything. We decided to push anyway and this is where Juju's pushing and crowning classes became so important. I visualised that coffee plunger and in doing so I could concentrate on bearing down from the top of my belly, right from my ribcage down. Having learned from Juju the physicality of how the muscles work, and what the actual pushing does, I was able to be in touch with my body even though I couldn't feel a thing.

In the end, after about 45 minutes of pushing, the baby needed to be suctioned but before we knew it our baby boy arrived. My husband and I had just been through one of the most magical, emotional, physically trying adventures we could ever imagine having. We worked through each contraction together, a team, breathing together, moving together, counting together, shouting together, laughing together, crying together. When one of us would wane, the other would be there for them. We were going through this as a team. And now I had my baby boy in my arms. It felt fantastic. We were so proud of ourselves and of him. Our experience was beyond anything we could have imagined. It brought us closer than we ever knew was possible. Every day we look at our son and remember how he came into the world. We know we would never have experienced it in the way we did without Juju.

As I write this we are awaiting the birth of our second child with great anticipation. When Juju and I set out to write this book our aim was to pass on to you the knowledge of what your body and your mind are capable of, and to inspire you to give it a try. If I had opted right away for an epidural for the birth of my first son I would never have felt what my body and my baby could do. I am still in awe of what we achieved! Like me, you are about to experience one of nature's most precious gifts. And I hope, like me, you will be amazed and surprised by what you are capable of. There is nothing more precious than our children, and the bonding that can be achieved by giving it a go is amazing.

ACKNOWLEDGEMENTS

Thank you ...

Dr Keith Hartman has been telling me to write this book for years. For over 30 years he has had the integrity and vision to encourage, support and offer wise counsel to an obstetric physiotherapist always wanting to push the envelope of ideas and concepts in antenatal education. My love, gratitude and respect are infinite. Sarah and I particularly thank him for his support with this project.

Thank you to The Mater Hospital, North Sydney. Over the years the hospital has been superb to both of us in different ways.

The Crows Nest Community Centre also provided the location for our class photography and we are indebted to Bonds Clothing for providing their beautiful sportswear. We thank them both.

We would also like to thank Exercise Australia, Quintessence Homewares, Abby McGrath, Yanni Hatsatouris, Marina Sundin, Heidi Sundin, David Catterns QC, Natasha Severino, David Keough, Carol O'Hare, Ian Phillip and Carol Fallows. They have all provided help and support in different ways and it is very much appreciated.

Ian Lovegreen has been doing the photography for my practice for over 25 years. His humour, friendship and professionalism are greatly appreciated.

Thank you to the men and women from my classes who have featured in the photography throughout the Australian edition of the book, and so generously contributed their labour excerpts and stories. We also thank all of their partners and other support people who are not named, yet provided the vital teamwork during childbirth. Without exception each woman states she could not have done it without her partner. For privacy and to protect anonymity we have used only the first names of the women and men who have made contributions to the text. Every effort has been made to contact the individual copyright holders of this material but it has not been possible in all cases. However, we thank and acknowledge them all.

We have been proud to have been part of the Allen and Unwin Publishing team, working with publisher Jude McGee, senior editor Joanne Holliman, designer Robyn Latimer and illustrator Jan Garben. Our literary agent Fiona Inglis from Curtis Brown has been our 'rock' every step of the way. Thank you.

Last but not least, I wish to thank all the men and women who have passed through my practice over the last 35 and more years for their contributions to the content of this book. I am proud of all of you. Thank you for what you have taught me. I carry your stories with me each time I give a class.

Copyright

INDEX

abdominal muscles, role during the pushing stage 172
activity plus focus 1–2
adrenalin
  as motivator 271–3
  effects on endorphin release 28
  effects on oxytocin release 28
  response to labour pain 21–2, 23
  response to threat or crisis 21–2, 23
  utilising adrenalin for action 27–31
  working off excess 8–9
amygdala 7

backache labour see posterior backache labour
Bannister, Roger 37–8
breath, internalising during the pushing stage 173–4, 187
breathing and vocalising 51–85
  benefits of rhythmic activity 51
  changing attitudes 52, 54–8
  do it your way 63
  effects of holding your breath 51
  example of use through first stage of labour 60–2
  externalising stress 64
  importance of letting go 55
  inhibitions about vocalisation 52–3, 84
  learning 'the breathing' 53–8
  matching the pain 60
  physiology of breathing in labour 58–60
  Sound Blocks Pain class 52
  stress and pain release 58–60
  thoughts on pain mastery 71

see also breathing skills; vocalising skills
breathing skills 65–8
  add a 'yes' 65–6
  blow it all away 66–7
  listening to your sound 65
  'open' up 66
  too soon to push 67
  watching your breath 65
  working the words 66
  caution, hyperventilation 68
  guidelines for breathing 67
  Sarah's story 72–8
  see also breathing and vocalisation

caesarean, possible reasons for 240
calm birthing 57
cervix, process of dilation 24–6
childbirth DVDs 171
contractions see uterine contractions
control over labour pain 4–5 see also labour pain
cord, cutting 206
crowning 189–206
  definition 189
  effects on the perineum 191–3
  episiotomy 190, 193
  perineal massage 190–1
  physiology 191–2
  positions for giving birth 192
  preparation for 189–91
  preparing the pelvic floor muscles 190–1
  preparing the perineum 190–1

what to do during crowning 192–3
crowning exercises 193–200
  panting 193–4
  the grapefruit and the sock 195–6
  tissue paper imagery 194–5
  watching yourself 196
  Sarah's story 197–200

diaphragm, role during the pushing
  stage 172–6

emotions after the birth 205–6
endorphins 8–9
  effects of adrenalin 28
  increasing 24
epidural
  possible reasons for 240
  pushing stage with 169, 170, 176
  use in posterior backache labour 229
episiotomy 190, 193

Farrugia, Amelia 84
fear/freeze reflex 6–7, 29
fight/flight reflex 21, 29
first stage of labour 5
first stage of labour, skills
  breathing and vocalising 51–85
  keywords 139–66
  movement 17–50
  practice skills 211–15
  stress balls 113–38
  visualisation 87–112
foetus ejection reflex 169, 179

general adaptation syndrome 21
gentle birthing 57
Goddard, Trisha 114

hand activity *see* stress balls
healthy pain 6–7, 22–3
hypnobirthing 52, 57

instinctive behaviours during labour
  4–5, 139–40
intellectual control, optimal functioning
  level 148–9

Kemp, Peter 154
keyword skills 149–60
  coming to your senses 152
  extra images for you both 153–4
  extras for your partner 153
  key words for pain and stress 150
  mantras for stress balls 150
  moving words 152
  see the numbers 154
  smell deep 151
  tension release 152–3
  vocalisation partners 153
  watching the birth process 151–2
  what do you see? 151
  partner's role 154–5
  Sarah's story 156–60
keywords 139–66
  choice of words 141–9
  effects of focusing on words 141–2
  focus away from the pain 146–9
  'Go' 29
  how to use them 146–9
  matching the pain 144
  optimal functioning level 148–9
  physiological effects 141–2
  reframing negative thoughts 147–8
  swearing 142–3
  word options 143–4

labour kit bag, Sarah's suggestions 220
labour pain
  adrenalin response 21–2, 23
  body's natural chemical help 8–9
  control over labour pain 4–5
  dilation of the cervix 24–6
  fear/freeze reflex 6–7
  healthy pain 6–7, 22–3

healthy responses to 5–7
location of the pain 26–7
match the pain 30
pain-free leg activity 23–4
pain-reducing adaptation 26–7
response to threat or crisis 21–2, 23
stages of 5–6
see also first stage of labour, skills;
   posterior backache labour; second
   stage of labour, skills
labour process
  importance of education 9–10
  using birth skills 10–13
  see also first stage of labour; second
   stage of labour; third stage of labour
Lamaze method 52
leg activity to control pain 23–4, 27–31
  see also movement
Legs for Labour class 19–20

medical help 239–63
  possible reasons for a caesarean 240
  possible reasons for an epidural 240
motivation and birth skills 265–74
  proactivity, possibility and potential
   266–7
  ten ways to motivate yourself 268–70
  your objective 270–1
movement 17–50
  leg activity to control pain 23–4
  Legs for Labour class 19–20
  pain-free rhythmic activity 27–31
  response to threat or crisis 21–2
  using adrenalin 27–31
movement skills 32–47
  calf sliding 34
  fit ball bounce 35–6
  floor mat marching 33–4
  pacing the floor 33
  palms on thighs 35
  rhythmic stepping 33
  rock and sway 32

wall sliding 35
water stomping 34
  cautions 37
  partner's role 36
  Sarah's story 38–47

natural chemical help during labour
   8–9

optimal functioning level 148–9
oxytocin release 8
  effects of adrenalin 28

pain mastery, thoughts on 71 *see also*
   labour pain
partner's role
  guidelines for vocalisation 69
  helping with posterior backache
   labour 233–4
  keyword skills 154–5
  movement skills 36
  stress ball skills 124
  understanding about physiology 31
  visualisation exercises 103
pelvic floor exercise 210
pelvic floor muscles
  preparing for crowning 190–1
  relaxing during pushing stage 172
Pemberton, Rex 271
perineal massage 190–1
perineum
  effects of crowning 191–3
  preparing for crowning 190–1
Pert, Candace 8
Pilates 52
placenta, delivery of 5, 205
positions for giving birth 192
posterior backache labour
  indications and what to do 230–2
  questions when labour starts 230–2
  use of an epidural 229
  what it means 223–6

what to do during posterior labour
227–30
what to expect 226–7
what your partner can do to help 233–4
practice
labour objectives 217–18
losing inhibitions 209
make sure you know your skills 209–21
mental practice and imagery 221
pelvic floor exercise 210
think 'solution' 209–10
practice skills for first stage 211–15
in the all-fours position 214–15
kneeling 214
lying down 215
while sitting 213–14
while standing 212–13
practice skills for transition 215–18
pre-labour 5
premature pushing urge 180
preparation
medical help if you need it 239–63
motivation and birth skills 265–74
posterior backache labour 223–38
Sarah's top-ten tips 218–19
using a range of activities 57
pushing 169–88
active pushing 169–70
embarrassment and inhibitions 175
foetus ejection reflex 169–70
internalising the breath 173–4, 187
lack of pain during 170–1
physiology 172–4
premature pushing urge 180
pushing urge 172
role of the abdominal muscles 172
role of the diaphragm 172–6
role of the uterus 172–6
urge to bear down 172
use of imagery 169–70
what to do 174–6
when it starts 170–1
with an epidural 169, 170, 176

pushing skills 176–83
the bottom end 177
the coffee plunger 176–7, 178–80
caution 178
Sarah's story 181–3
visualisation for pushing 177–8

reframing negative thoughts 147–8

Sarah's labour kit bag 220
Sarah's story 2–4
breathing and vocalising 72–8
crowning exercises 197–200
keyword skills 156–60
movement skills 38–47
pushing skills 181–3
stress ball skills 126–32
the bigger picture 275–81
top-ten tips 218–19
visualisation exercises 104–8
Sarkisian, Yurik 209–10
second stage of labour 5–6
childbirth DVDs 171
second stage of labour, skills
crowning 189–206
pushing 169–88
sense of smell, utilising 93
sense of touch, utilising 93
Shaw, Margaret 273–4
Singleman, Glen 272
skills *see* first stage of labour, skills;
second stage of labour, skills
Spencer, Danielle 53
stress, utilising adrenalin for action
27–31
stress ball skills 120–32
a climbing bang 123
breathe and squeeze 123
colour awareness 121
countdown 123
listen closely 121
rhythmic moves 121

see it in your mind 122
seeing red 122
tune in 123
cautions 123
partner's role 124
points to remember 125
Sarah's story 126–32
stress balls 113–38
  active hands block pain 114–15
  objectives of stress ball activity
    118–19
  physiology of hand activity 115–16
  ways to use them 117
  working in different positions 120
Sutherland, Joan 19–20
Swan, Heather 272

ten ways to motivate yourself 268–70
the bigger picture, Sarah's story 275–81
The Little Prince 71
third stage of labour 5
  cutting the cord 206
  delivery of the placenta 205
  emotions after the birth 205–6
transition, practice for 215–18

urge to bear down 172
uterine contractions
  body's natural chemical help 8–9
  dilation of the cervix 24–6
  healthy pain 6–7, 22–3
  internal processes 24–6
  location of the pain 26–7
  muscle fatigue 22–3
  pain-reducing adaptation 26–7
  see also first stage of labour; second
    stage of labour; third stage of labour
uterus, role during the pushing stage
    172–6

vagina
  preparation for crowning 190–1

stretching during crowning 191–3
visualisation 87–112
  and sense of smell 93
  and sense of touch 93
  daydreaming 89–90
  diversity of ways to use 108–11
  for pushing 177–8
  how to use during stages of labour
    92–5
  ideas for images to focus on 90–2
  physiology of vision 95–6
  putting it into practice 96–7
  what it involves 88–92
visualisation exercises 97–108
  blowing out the candle 102
  colour beats 100
  count up, count down 102
  flower power 100
  fragrant bubbles 101–2
  imagining the unseen 98–9
  sights and sounds 101
  turn on the tap 103
  walking together 99
  waterfall 100–1
  partner's role 103
  Sarah's story 104–8
  your action plan 98
vocalising skills 68–78
  make it a team effort 70
  see a message 69
  send it out 70
  sound for transition 70
  the 'Aahh' sound 69
  think a message 69–70
  throw away those inhibitions 70
  vary the rhythm 69
  guidelines for the partner 69
  guidelines for the woman 68
  Sarah's story 72–8
  see also breathing and vocalisation

yoga breathing 52, 53, 57

Pregnancy and birth resources by Juju Sundin

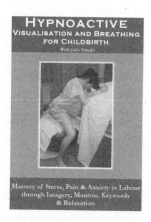
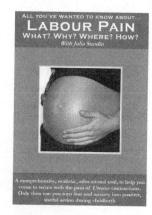
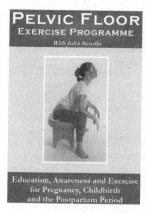
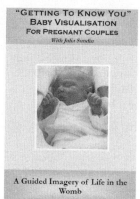
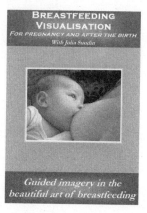
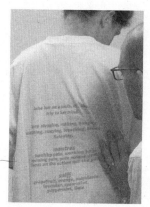